Nutrition
A Handbook for Community Nurses

JUDY BUTTRISS PhD, SRD, RPHNutr
Science Director, British Nutrition Foundation

AMANDA WYNNE BSc, MSc, PGDipDiet, SRD

and

SARA STANNER BSc(Hons), MSc, RPHNutr
Nutrition Scientist British Nutrition Foundation

SERIES EDITOR
MARILYN EDWARDS BSc(Hons), SRN, FETC
Specialist Practitioner, General Practice Nursing, Bilbrook Medical
Centre, Staffordshire

W
WHURR PUBLISHERS
LONDON AND PHILADELPHIA

© 2001 Whurr Publishers Ltd
First published 2001
by Whurr Publishers Ltd
19b Compton Terrace
London N1 2UN England and
325 Chestnut Street, Philadelphia PA 19106 USA

Reprinted 2001

British Library Cataloguing in Publication Data

A catalogue record for this book
is available from the British Library.

ISBN 1 86156 216 0

Printed and bound in the UK by Athenaeum Press Ltd,
Gateshead, Tyne & Wear.

Contents

Series Preface

This series of handbooks has been devised to help community nurses answer commonly asked questions. Many of the questions are asked by patients, others by colleagues. The books have been written by specialists, and although they are not intended as full clinical texts, they are fully referenced from current evidence to validate the content. The purpose of each handbook is to provide 'facts at the fingertips', so that trawling through textbooks is not needed. This is achieved through the question and answer format, with cross referencing between sections. Where further information may be required, the reader is referred to specific texts. Many patients want some control over their illnesses, and use the internet to access information. The useful address sections include website addresses to share with both patients and colleagues.

It is hoped that these handy reference books will answer most everyday questions. If there are areas which you feel have been neglected, please let us know for future editions.

Mandy Edwards

Introduction

It has long been recognised that achieving optimal health involves more than just preventing disease. To achieve optimal health status, and reduce chances of early death and ill-health, it is important to follow a healthy balanced diet, to stay fit and active, to avoid smoking and to moderate alcohol consumption.

The government recognised, in *Saving Lives: Our Healthier Nation* (Department of Health, 1999) (see page 2), that public health is an important consideration and that nurses, midwives and health visitors can play a crucial role in promoting good health. Relevant aspects of this strategy paper are discussed below, and a strategy is being developed, which will help develop the public health aspects of the role of nurses (National Health Service Executive, 1999). There is clearly a key role for nurses and other health professionals to promote positive and practical dietary messages, to help people to improve the balance of their nutritional intake and to implement a regimen of physical activity, in order to optimise health and well-being. In the future, there may also be a new role developed for nurses, namely specialist in public health, i.e. equivalent to a medically qualified consultant in terms of status.

Background

The importance of promoting good health through nutrition was recognised in Government policy in 1992, when the *Health of the Nation* White Paper (Department of Health, 1992) was launched. This paper set out plans to 'add life to years and years to life'. This strategy was based on five priority areas: cancer; coronary heart disease (CHD) and stroke; accidents; mental illness; and HIV/AIDS and sexual health. It was recognised that, in relation to cancer, CHD and stroke, nutrition could have an impact and as such a number of diet and nutrition targets were set. These were to:

- reduce fat intake to 35% of food energy
- reduce saturated fatty acid intake to no more than 11% of food energy
- reduce obesity to 6% in men and 8% in women
- reduce the proportion of men drinking over 21 units a week and of women drinking over 14 units a week by 30% (to 18% of men and 7% of women). (These guidelines have subsequently been revised – see Q1.6.)

There was also a recommendation to reduce mean systolic blood pressure by 5 mmHg by the year 2005. A Nutrition Task Force was set up to look at ways of implementing these targets: its report, *Eat Well*, was published in 1994 (Department of Health, 1994a).

Current Health Targets – *Saving Lives: Our Healthier Nation*

The latest Government White Paper on this subject, *Saving Lives: Our Healthier Nation* (Department of Health, 1999), was launched in July 1999. This report identified as its key aims the improvement of the health of everyone, and the health of the worst off in particular. The following are the four key areas targeted for action:

1. Cancer: to reduce death rates in the under-75s by at least one fifth.
2. Coronary heart disease and stroke: to reduce death rates in the under-75s by at least two-fifths.
3. Accidents: to reduce death by at least one fifth and serious injury by at least one tenth.
4. Mental illness: to reduce death rate from suicide and undetermined injury by at least one fifth.

The White Paper recognises that understanding how people live their lives, what they eat, how active they are and whether they smoke is central to improving health. The Government recognises the importance of physical activity and the White Paper refers to plans to put together a strategy that will ensure wide-ranging sports and leisure opportunities at a local level, the promotion of exercise on prescription and the development of specific sports programmes to encourage activity among people with stress, obesity and diabetes.

It is also recognised by the government that diet is central to health throughout life. Consumption of plenty of fruit, vegetables and cereals is recommended, along with the need to moderate or reduce consumption of foods providing large amounts of fat and/or salt. No specific targets on diet or nutrition are given, however, in the 1999 document, although subsequently plans have been outlined in the NHS Plan (Department of Health 2000a), for example the free school fruit scheme for 4–6 year olds (see Department of Health 2000b). There is also concern expressed about people living in deprived neighbourhoods, where there may be difficulty in reaching shops that sell affordable foods (see below).

Nutrition-related recommendations made in the White Paper are as follows. There is recognition of the need for the following:

- Further measures to improve the nutrition provided at school
- A comprehensive review of the common agricultural policy's impact on health and inequalities in health
- Policies that increase the availability and accessibility of foodstuffs to supply an adequate and affordable diet
- Policies that improve the health and nutrition of women of child-bearing age and their children, with priority given to the elimination of food poverty and prevention and reduction of obesity
- Policies that increase the prevalence of breast-feeding.

Nutritional Issues Highlighted in *Saving Lives: Our Healthier Nation*

The following are all areas highlighted by the Government in their recent strategy document.

Salt

The Government has begun a series of meetings with the food industry to explore ways of reducing the salt content of processed foods. A number of major retailers have already taken action to reduce the salt content of their own-brand products. Around 90%

of the salt we eat is derived from processed foods. Looking for lower salt options in the supermarket, avoidance of adding salt during cooking and use of alternative seasonings at the table can help to reduce salt intake. It is important, however, to ensure that nutritional messages are placed in context. It is recognised in the report that salt is not the only factor that affects blood pressure. Reducing excess alcohol intake and increasing physical activity are also highlighted as being important.

Practical advice for those with high blood pressure should focus on diet and lifestyle. Maintenance of a body weight within the desirable range should be promoted, along with regular physical activity and adherence to sensible drinking guidelines (no more than two to three drinks a day for women and no more than three or four drinks a day for men). In dietary terms, excess salt intake should be avoided and consumption of fruit and vegetables encouraged to provide potassium. Low-fat dairy products should also be promoted as a useful source of calcium, which may also beneficially affect blood pressure. For further information, see Q4.2.

Obesity

There is no specific target given for tackling obesity in *Saving Lives: Our Healthier Nation*. The targets set in the previous health strategy, *The Health of the Nation*, to reduce obesity incidence to 6% of men and 8% of women, were very ambitious. The latest figures on obesity (BMI > 30) show that it has now risen to 17% in men and 20% in women in England (Department of Health, 1999). Altogether, 62% of men and 53% of women can now be classed as overweight (BMI > 25). The Government states in *Saving Lives: Our Healthier Nation* that the provision of information on healthy eating and the importance of physical activity will help prevent obesity. It may be, however, that a more clearly defined strategy is needed to begin to tackle this problem. A major review of obesity, published by the British Nutrition Foundation (1999a), suggested key action for policy-makers. This might include fundamental changes in legislation, e.g. new legislation to clamp down on miracle weight-loss cures that undermine the efforts of reputable healthcare professionals and new transport policies that promote increased levels of physical activity.

The relationship between obesity and health is discussed more fully in Q4.4–4.12. Specific issues relating to obesity are discussed throughout the book and a Government framework for tackling obesity at local level can be found in the National Service Framework for CHD (Department of Health 2000c).

Breast-feeding

The benefits of breast-feeding are recognised by the Government, which is aiming to increase the prevalence of breast-feeding, especially in areas of the country where breast-feeding rates are lowest. For more information see Q3.21–3.34. There are numerous benefits associated with breast-feeding (see Q3.24). As well as being a complete nutrient source, breast milk has anti-infective properties and contains a variety of enzymes, growth factors, hormones, nutrient-binding proteins and non-absorbable carbohydrates. Breast-feeding may also help in the development of a warm mother/child relationship.

Importance of good nutrition for schoolchildren

High on the Government's agenda is the need to focus on the health of Britain's schoolchildren. The implementation of good habits in childhood is important for the future health of the population. Over the last 50 years, there has been a change in emphasis in relation to concerns about schoolchildren's diets. Historically, the focus was on the adequate provision of nutrients, but providing adequate dietary balance is now viewed as the main priority. The National Diet and Nutrition Survey of young people (aged 4–18 years) is the most detailed survey yet to be undertaken in this age group in Britain (Gregory et al., 2000). This survey demonstrates that, although vitamin intakes are generally adequate, a sizeable proportion of children, particularly older girls, may have inadequate intakes of some minerals. Also, there is a high intake of saturated fatty acids, non-milk extrinsic sugars and salt among many children. Moreover, with the exception of the youngest children (4–6 years), young people in Britain are largely inactive. Clearly, these findings are worthy of our attention because poor eating and physical activity habits in childhood can store up problems for later life, particularly in relation to obesity, heart disease, diabetes, osteoporosis and cancer.

There is clear evidence from the survey to justify the Government's concern about the diets of children living in households where there is relative poverty. In particular, boys in households in receipt of benefits seem to have lower energy intakes and poorer-quality diets (Gregory et al., 2000). The independent report to the Government on health inequalities from Professor Acheson indicated that one in three of Britain's children lives in poverty and, in 1996, 2.2 million children in Britain were in families receiving income support (Acheson, 1998). This report highlighted the important role of education in influencing health inequalities and providing children with practical and social skills, including budgeting and cooking. The Government's Healthy Schools programme is aimed at creating a healthy ethos in schools. This remit includes promoting good nutrition and the acquisition of cooking skills, as well as increased levels of physical activity. There are also plans to re-establish national nutritional standards for school meals, which came into force in April 2001.

A number of initiatives are under way to improve the nutrition of schoolchildren and their awareness of healthy eating, including school breakfast schemes, 'healthy' tuck shops and the development of 'Wired for Health' – a website for teachers providing health information to support the National Curriculum. Pilots for a scheme to provide 4–6 year olds with free fruit at school, are underway with a view to implementation by 2004 (Department of Health 2000b). For further information, see Q3.59–3.76. The government has also published a sports strategy which aims to encourage physical activity among children by providing after school activities for all pupils and establishing school sport co-ordinators in communities of greatest need (for further details see Sports England website).

Shopping access and food deserts

With a key emphasis placed on inequalities in health, the Government plans to tackle the 'food desert' issue. This is a term used to describe the situation where people living in deprived neighbourhoods are unable to access the out-of-town large supermarkets that sell affordable and healthy foods, because of lack of car ownership or poor public transport, and hence are obliged to shop locally in smaller shops that offer less choice at higher prices (see Q3.103). It is hoped that, by developing policies that improve shopping access, a healthy range of foods will become available to everyone and this will be accompanied by improved nutritional intake. The reintroduction of home delivery services is a simple way to increase shopping access.

Folic acid

All women of child-bearing age embarking on a pregnancy are now advised to supplement their dietary intake with a daily 400 µg folic acid supplement, because this has been shown to reduce the chance of a neural tube defect (NTD) birth dramatically (see Q2.17 and Q3.2). The Government's advisory committee (COMA) report on folate/folic acid recommended the universal fortification of flour at 240 µg/100 g in food products as consumed, and estimated that this may reduce the risk of NTDs by around 40% (Department of Health, 2000a). A Government consultation on the issue of fortification took place during 2000 (see Q 1.12).

Five-a-day campaign for fruit and vegetables

To improve dietary balance and to help reduce the risk of several chronic diseases occurring prematurely, an increase in intake of fruit and vegetables to a minimum of five portions (various different types) per day has been recommended (see Q1.2). Various national and local initiatives are already under way to help promote this positive message.

Nutrition and older people

A recent Government's advisory committee (COMA) report on bone health (Department of Health, 1998a) and a national survey of the diet and nutritional status of older people have both identified the need for greater awareness of the importance of adequate vitamin D (via sunlight or the diet), particularly for older people; they also identified the need for continued fortification of specific foods with vitamin D (margarines, low fat spreads) and calcium (all flour except wholemeal, including bread flour). Other nutritional concerns identified in the survey of older people included: poor folate status and poor dental health, particularly in institutionalised older people (see Q3.112).

Contents

This book has been written to provide community nurses with basic and topical practical information on various aspects of nutrition, to help in the provision of comprehensive dietary advice and information.

Chapter 1 discusses healthy eating and nutrition and includes an overview of the current healthy eating guidelines, dietary reference values and basic information on macronutrients, vitamins and minerals. Chapter 2 explains the role of the different nutrients and describes their relationships in promoting health. Chapter 3 outlines the differing needs and health concerns of various groups in the population, including pregnant women, infants, schoolchildren, adolescents and elderly people.

The importance of nutrition in disease prevention is examined in Chapter 4, with a look at practical dietary advice for prevention and treatment of diet-related diseases. The aetiology and medical management of disease are not discussed, although mention is made where appropriate.

Issues in the media tend to provoke controversial discussion. Chapter 5 looks at some of the common media stories and puts these topical issues into a scientific perspective. This chapter also includes a short section on food hygiene, which offers important advice for minimising the risk of food poisoning.

It is important for the reader to be able to assess the validity of new research. Chapter 6 offers the basic tools needed for critical appraisal of new scientific studies. The roles of the state-registered dietitian and the registered public health nutritionist are often misunderstood, and are clarified in this chapter. A list of useful addresses can also be found at the end of the book.

The book has been written in a question and answer format, to enable the reader to cross-reference topics. There will inevitably be some overlap of topics throughout the book; this overlap will reinforce essential points.

Chapter 1
A Healthy Diet

It is now well recognised that a 'healthy' diet should contain an adequate supply of all the essential nutrients to prevent deficiency, as well as providing the right balance of these nutrients to protect against nutrition-related health problems. This chapter describes current guidelines and provides practical advice to ensure that the diet is meeting both of these criteria.

Q1.1 So what exactly is a healthy diet?

The answer is one that provides all the nutrients required by the body, in the right proportions. Traditionally, nutritional recommendations were based on preventing deficiency of a nutrient. Today, thinking has moved on and, as nutritional science develops, recommendations are refined and updated in order to promote optimal health. For example, the reference nutrient intake for folate/folic acid in women is 200 μg/day. It is now known, however, that an additional 400 μg/day of folic acid taken before conception and during the first 12 weeks of pregnancy will help prevent neural tube defects (see Q2.17 and Q3.2). Furthermore, increased intakes of folic acid can lower blood levels of homocysteine, an amino acid thought to be linked to coronary heart disease (CHD). However, it is not yet clear whether or not, by taking extra folic acid, the prevalence of CHD can be reduced (Department of Health, 2000d). It is, therefore, clear that intakes of folate/folic acid over and above levels that prevent deficiency will be beneficial in some population groups.

Q1.2 How is diet related to health?

Many modern diseases are linked to diet to some extent, most notably CHD, stroke, some cancers, diabetes and obesity. Optimising nutritional intake can help reduce premature morbidity and mortality from these diseases (see Chapter 4). It is important to consider both the proportion of energy derived from the macronutrients (protein, fat and carbohydrate) and the intakes of vitamins, minerals and dietary fibre. In addition, there is growing evidence that a number of substances found in fruit and vegetables, sometimes called phytochemicals, may be important in promoting good health (see Q2.9 and Q5.9). These substances are the subject of a current British Nutrition Foundation Task Force, the report of which is due to be published in 2001.

Dietary Reference Values

Q1.3 What are dietary reference values?

Recommendations for nutrient intakes in the UK have existed for over 30 years. Recommended intakes for nutrients were published by the DHSS in 1969 and recommended daily amounts (RDAs) were published by the DHSS in 1979. These values were designed to assess the nutritional adequacy of the diets of groups of people. More recently, a range of figures has been calculated that can be used to assess both the diets of groups and, with care and expertise, individuals. These are called dietary reference values (DRVs) and were published by the Department of Health in 1991. The term 'reference' was used in the hope that the figures would be used as a general point of reference, rather than as a definitive recommendation. The relationship between the various reference values is shown in Figure 1.1. All the recommendations are intended to apply to healthy people.

Energy, protein, vitamins and minerals

Estimated average requirement (EAR)

This is the estimate of the average requirement or need for food energy or a nutrient. Some people will need more than the average and some people will need less. For energy intakes, only EARs exist (Table 1.1).

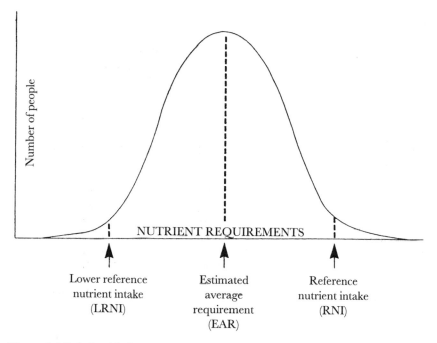

Figure 1.1 Relationship between various reference values.

Reference nutrient intake (RNI)

This is an amount of a nutrient that is enough for almost every individual, even those with high needs, i.e. the amount of a nutrient that is enough for 97% of the population. If an individual is regularly consuming the RNI, that individual is unlikely to be deficient in the nutrient in question. RNIs for vitamins and minerals are shown in Tables 1.2 and 1.3.

Lower reference nutrient intake (LRNI)

This is the amount of a nutrient that is enough for a small number of people with low needs, i.e. the amount of a nutrient that is enough for just 3% of the population. If an individual is regularly consuming less than the LRNI, he or she will almost certainly be deficient. Tables 1.4 and 1.5 show the LRNIs for vitamins and minerals.

Safe intake

This is a term used to indicate the recommended intake of a nutrient for which there is not enough information available to give a range of

Table 1.1 Estimated average requirements (EARs) for energy

Age	EARs MJ/day (kcal/day)	
	Males	Females
0–3 months	2.28 (545)	2.16 (515)
4–6 months	2.89 (690)	2.69 (645)
7–9 months	3.44 (825)	3.20 (765)
10–12 months	3.85 (920)	3.61 (865)
1–3 years	5.15 (1230)	4.86 (1165)
4–6 years	7.16 (1715)	6.46 (1545)
7–10 years	8.24 (1970)	7.28 (1740)
11–14 years	9.27 (2220)	7.92 (1845)
15–18 years	11.51 (2755)	8.83 (2110)
19–50 years	10.60 (2550)	8.10 (1940)
51–59 years	10.60 (2550)	8.00 (1900)
60–64 years	9.93 (2380)	7.99 (1900)
65–74 years	9.71 (2330)	7.96 (1900)
75+ years	8.77 (2100)	7.61 (1810)
Pregnancy		+0.80[a] (200)
Lactation		
1 month		+1.90 (450)
2 months		+2.20 (530)
3 months		+2.40 (570)
4–6 months (group 1)[b]		+2.00 (480)
4–6 months (group 2)[b]		+2.40 (570)
>6 months (group 1)		+1.00 (240)
> 6 months (group 2)		+2.30 (550)

[a]Last trimester only.
[b]Group 1: women who exclusively breast-feed until 3–4 months and then progressively introduce weaning foods. Group 2: women who provide breast milk as the primary source of nourishment for 6 months or more.
Source: Department of Health (1991).

values. A safe intake is judged to be adequate for almost everyone's needs, but is not so high as to cause undesirable effects (Table 1.6).

Dietary reference values (DRVs)

This is a general term that covers all the other terms, i.e. RNI, EAR, LRNI and safe intake.

Table 1.2 Reference nutrient intakes for vitamins

Age	Thiamin (mg/day)	Riboflavin (mg/day)	Niacin (nicotinic acid equivalent) (mg/day)	Vitamin B6 (mg/day)[a]	Vitamin B12 (µg/day)	Folate (µg/day)[b]	Vitamin C (mg/day)	Vitamin A (µg/day)	Vitamin D (µg/day)
0–3 months	0.2	0.4	3	0.2	0.3	50	25	350	8.5
4–6 months	0.2	0.4	3	0.2	0.3	50	25	350	8.5
7–9 months	0.2	0.4	4	0.3	0.4	50	25	350	7
10–12 months	0.3	0.4	5	0.4	0.4	50	25	350	7
1–3 years	0.5	0.6	8	0.7	0.5	70	30	400	7
4–6 years	0.7	0.8	11	0.9	0.8	100	30	400	–
7–10 years	0.7	1.0	12	1.0	1.0	150	30	500	–
Males									
11–14 years	0.9	1.2	15	1.2	1.2	200	35	600	–
15–18 years	1.1	1.3	18	1.5	1.5	200	40	700	–
19–50 years	1.0	1.3	17	1.4	1.5	200	40	700	–
50+ years	0.9	1.3	16	1.4	1.5	200	40	700	d
Females									
1–14 years	0.7	1.1	12	1.0	1.2	200	35	600	–
15–18 years	0.8	1.1	14	1.2	1.5	200	40	600	–
19–50 years	0.8	1.1	13	1.2	1.5	200	40	600	–
50+ years	0.8	1.1	12	1.2	1.5	200	40	600	d

(contd)

Table 1.2 (contd)

Age	Thiamin (mg/day)	Riboflavin (mg/day)	Niacin (nicotinic acid equivalent) (mg/day)	Vitamin B6 (mg/day)[a]	Vitamin B12 (µg/day)	Folate (µg/day)[b]	Vitamin C (mg/day)	Vitamin A (µg/day)	Vitamin D (µg/day)
Pregnancy	+0.1[c]	+0.3	[c]	[c]	[c]	+100	+10	+100	10
Lactation									
0–4 months	+0.2	+0.5	+2	[c]	+0.5	+60	+30	+350	10
4+ months	+0.2	+0.5	+2	[c]	+0.5	+60	+30	+350	10

[a]Based on protein providing 14.7% of EAR for energy.
[b]A 400 µg/day supplement has subsequently been recommended for all women of child-bearing age embarking on a pregnancy, to be continued until week 12 of pregnancy.
[c]No increment.
[d]After age 65 the RNI is 10 mg/day for men and women.
[e]For last trimester only.
Source: Department of Health (1991).

Table 1.3 Reference nutrient intakes for minerals[b]

Age	Calcium (mg/day)	Phosphorus[a] (mg/day)	Magnesium (mg/day)	Sodium (mg/day)[b]	Potassium (mg/day)[c]	Chloride (mg/day)[d]	Iron (mg/day)	Zinc (mg/day)	Copper (mg/day)	Selenium (µg/day)	Iodine (µg/day)
0–3 months	525	400	55	210	800	320	1.7	4.0	0.2	10	50
4–6 months	525	400	60	280	850	400	4.3	4.0	0.3	13	60
7–9 months	525	400	75	320	700	500	7.8	5.0	0.3	10	60
10–12 months	525	400	80	350	700	500	7.8	5.0	0.3	10	60
1–3 years	350	270	85	500	800	800	6.9	5.0	0.4	15	70
4–6 years	450	350	120	700	1100	1100	6.1	6.5	0.6	20	100
7–10 years	550	450	200	1200	2000	1800	8.7	7.0	0.7	30	110
Males											
11–14 years	1000	775	280	1600	3100	2500	11.3	9.0	0.8	45	130
15–18 years	1000	775	300	1600	3500	2500	11.3	9.5	1.0	70	140
19–50 years	700	550	300	1600	3500	2500	8.7	9.5	1.2	75	140
50+ years	700	550	300	1600	3500	2500	8.7	9.5	1.2	75	140
Females											
11–14 years	800	625	280	1600	3100	2500	14.8[e]	9.0	0.8	45	130
15–18 years	800	625	300	1600	3500	2500	14.8[e]	7.0	1.0	60	140
19–50 years	700	550	270	1600	3500	2500	14.8[e]	7.0	1.2	60	140
50+ years	700	550	270	1600	3500	2500	8.7	7.0	1.2	60	140

(contd)

Table 1.3 (contd)

Age	Calcium (mg/day)	Phosphorus[a] (mg/day)	Magnesium (mg/day)	Sodium (mg/day)[b]	Potassium (mg/day)[c]	Chloride (mg/day)[d]	Iron (mg/day)	Zinc (mg/day)	Copper (mg/day)	Selenium (µg/day)	Iodine (µg/day)
Pregnancy	f	f	f	f	f	f	f	f	f	f	f
Lactation											
0–4 months	+550	+440	+50	f	f	f	f	+6.0	+0.3	+15	f
4+ months	+550	+440	+50	f	f	f	f	+2.5	+0.3	+15	f

[a] Phosphorus RNI is set equal to calcium in molar terms.
[b] 1 mmol sodium = 23 mg.
[c] 1 mmol potassium = 39 mg.
[d] Corresponds to sodium 1 mmol = 35.5 mg.
[e] Insufficient for women with high menstrual losses where the most practical way of meeting iron requirements is to take iron supplements
[f] No increment.

Source: Department of Health (1991).

Table 1.4 Lower reference nutrient intakes for vitamins

Age	Thiamin (mg/day)	Riboflavin (mg/day)	Niacin (nicotinic acid equivalent) (mg/day)	Vitamin B6 (mg/day)	Vitamin B12 (µg/day)	Folate (µg/day)	Vitamin C (mg/day)	Vitamin A (µg/day) (retinol equivalents)	Vitamin D (µg/day)
0–3 months	0.2	0.2	4.4	3.5	0.1	30	6	150	–
4–6 months	0.2	0.2	4.4	3.5	0.1	30	6	150	–
7–9 months	0.2	0.2	4.4	6	0.25	30	6	150	–
10–12 months	0.2	0.2	4.4	8	0.25	30	6	150	–
1–3 years	0.23	0.3	4.4	11	0.3	35	8	200	–
4–6 years	0.23	0.4	4.4	11	0.5	50	8	200	–
7–10 years	0.23	0.5	4.4	11	0.6	75	8	250	–
Males									
11–14 years	0.23	0.8	4.4	11	0.8	100	9	250	–
15–18 years	0.23	0.8	4.4	11	1.0	100	10	300	–
19–50 years	0.23	0.8	4.4	11	1.0	100	10	300	–
50+ years	0.23	0.8	4.4	11	1.0	100	10	300	–
Females									
11–14 years	0.23	0.8	4.4	11	0.8	100	9	250	–
15–18 years	0.23	0.8	4.4	11	1.0	100	10	250	–
19–50 years	0.23	0.8	4.4	11	1.0	100	10	250	–
50+ years	0.23	0.8	4.4	11	1.0	100	10	250	–

(contd)

Table 1.4 (contd)

Age	Thiamin (mg/day)	Riboflavin (mg/day)	Niacin (nicotinic acid equivalent) (mg/day)	Vitamin B6 (mg/day)	Vitamin B12 (µg/day)	Folate (µg/day)	Vitamin C (mg/day)	Vitamin A (µg/day) (retinol equivalents)	Vitamin D (µg/day)
Pregnancy	a	—	a	a	a	—	—	—	—
Lactation									
0–4 months	a	—	—	a	—	—	—	—	—
4+ months	a	—	—	a	—	—	—	—	—

[a]No increment.

—, no LRNI set.

Source: Department of Health (1991).

Table 1.5 Lower reference nutrient intakes for minerals

Age	Calcium (mg/day)	Magnesium (mg/day)	Sodium (mg/day)	Potassium (mg/day)	Iron (mg/day)	Zinc (mg/day)	Selenium (µg/day)	Iodine (µg/day)
0–3 months	240	30	140	400	0.9	2.6	4	40
4–6 months	240	40	140	400	2.3	2.6	5	40
7–9 months	240	45	200	400	4.2	3.0	5	40
10–12 months	240	45	200	450	4.2	3.0	6	40
1–3 years	200	50	200	450	3.7	3.0	7	40
4–6 years	275	70	280	600	3.3	4.0	10	50
7–10 years	325	115	350	950	4.7	4.0	16	55
Males								
11–14 years	480	180	460	1600	6.1	5.3	25	65
15–18 years	480	190	575	2000	6.1	5.5	40	70
19–50 years	400	190	575	2000	4.7	5.5	40	70
50+ years	400	190	575	2000	4.7	5.5	40	70
Females								
11–14 years	450	180	460	1600	8.0	5.3	25	65
15–18 years	450	190	575	2000	8.0	4.0	40	70
19–50 years	400	150	575	2000	8.0	4.0	40	70
50+ years	400	150	575	2000	4.7	4.0	40	70
Pregnancy	[a]	[a]		—	—	[a]	[a]	[a]
Lactation							+15	[a]

[a]No increment.

Source: Department of Health (1991).

Table 1.6 Safe intakes

Nutrient	Safe intakes
Vitamins	
Pantothenic acid:	
adults	3–7 mg/day
infants	1.7 mg/day
Biotin	10–200 µg/day
Vitamin E:	
men	> 4 mg/day
women	> 3 mg/day
infants	0.4 mg/g polyunsaturated fatty acids
Vitamin K:	
adults	1 µg/kg per day
infants	10 µg/day
Minerals	
Manganese:	
adults	1.4 mg (26 µmol)/day
infants and children	16 mg (0.3 µmol)/day
Molybdenum:	
adults	50–400 µg/day
infants, children and adolescents	0.5–1.5 µg/kg per day
Chromium:	
adults	25 µg (0.5 mmol)/day
children and adolescents	0.1–1.0 µg (2–20 mmol)/kg per day
Fluoride (for infants only)	0.05 mg (3 µmol)/kg per day

Source: Department of Health (1991).

Fats, sugars and starches

These components of food are the main contributors towards energy requirements, unlike protein (which also contributes energy but is largely used for growth and tissue maintenance). Low intakes of fat, sugar and starches are not associated with deficiency symptoms and, as such, there can be no LRNI, EAR or RNI. There is, of course, a requirement for essential fatty acids but, if energy needs are met, this requirement will almost certainly be met. The proportions of these nutrients in the diet can have an impact on health, and DRVs are given in terms of recommended percentage contribution to dietary energy (Table 1.7).

Table 1.7 Dietary reference values for fat and carbohydrate for adults as a percentage of daily total energy intake (percentage of food energy given in brackets)

	Individual minimum	Population average	Individual maximum
Saturated fatty acids		10 (11)	
cis-polyunsaturated fatty acids	n-3 = 0.2 n-6 = 1.6	6 (6.5)	10
cis-monounsaturated fatty acids		12 (13)	
trans-fatty acids		2 (2)	
Total fatty acids		30 (32.5)	
Total fat		33 (35)	
Non-milk extrinsic sugars	0	10 (11)	
Intrinsic and milk sugars and starch		37 (39)	
Total carbohydrate		47 (50)	
Non-starch polysaccharide	12	18	24

Source: Department of Health (1991).

Dietary fibre

This is the term now used to replace 'roughage'. A dietary reference value of 18 g/day for adults has been given for non-starch polysaccharide (NSP), a means of assessing the fibre content of foods. This is based on an estimated desirable average intake. Corresponding figures do not exist for children, although it is recognised that they need proportionally less. Please note that a government decision made at the end of 2000 to change the method used to assess the fibre content of food, is likely to require derivation of a revised figure.

> Q1.4 Why are the DRVs sometimes different to the RDAs that appear on food labels?

There is often confusion between the DRVs and RDAs. Currently, RDA figures are specifically defined within the UK food labelling legislation, and differ slightly from the DRV recommendations. This is because the RDAs have been selected to be applicable across Europe, rather than in one country, and also to people in general, rather than a specific age/sex group. Where nutritional information is given on a food label, the RDA figure will be used by law. The

RDA is the value used as the basis of a 'minimum amount' declaration or a 'rich source' claim. Further information on RDAs can be found in the Food Labelling Regulations, 1996 (SI 1499, 1996).

The Components of a Healthy Diet

Q1.5 What are the components of a balanced diet?

A balanced diet is one that provides all the nutrients needed for health in the right proportions. In the UK, frank nutritional deficiency is, in general, uncommon. The major problem in the UK is dietary imbalance. Advice focuses on promoting the right balance of macronutrients, particularly carbohydrate and fat. It is recommended that half of our energy intake is provided by carbohydrate foods (mainly starchy foods); on average, energy intake from fat should be reduced to 35% and the remaining 15% should be provided by protein (see Table 1.7). Equally important is dietary variety, which helps achieve adequate intakes of micronutrients (vitamins and minerals) (see Tables 1.2 and 1.3).

Q1.6 What does this mean in practice, in terms of food?

In practical food terms, achieving a balanced diet is a matter of following a few basic guidelines. The Department of Health and the Ministry of Agriculture, Fisheries and Food (MAFF) have devised eight guidelines for a healthy diet, which are straightforward, and easy to follow and implement (Health Education Authority, 1995). These are as follows:

Enjoy your food

Food is one of the great pleasures in life and it is entirely possible for food to be healthy and enjoyable, despite misconceptions that prevail to the contrary. All the foods that are enjoyed by a particular individual can be included in a healthy diet (unless a particular medical condition prevails), as long as the overall balance of the diet is right.

Eat a variety of different foods

By including a variety of different foods in the diet, a wide variety of nutrients will be obtained and it will be unlikely that a deficiency of any particular nutrient will occur.

Eat the right amount to be a healthy weight

Obesity is increasing at a phenomenal rate in the UK, with one in five women now clinically obese and men not far behind (Department of Health, 1999). Given the associated health risks, most notably CHD, stroke, some cancers and diabetes, it is important to address this problem where necessary. Those who are clinically obese should try to lose weight gradually by eating sensibly and being physically active. Those within the ideal weight range should maintain their weight at this level (see Q4.5–4.12).

Eat plenty of foods rich in starch and fibre

Most of our dietary energy should be provided by starchy foods such as bread, rice, breakfast cereals, pasta and potatoes. Wholegrain varieties, which are higher in fibre, are the best choices. These foods should make up a large proportion of all main meals, and snacks such as toast, cereal or scones can also make a useful contribution to intake of starchy carbohydrate.

Eat plenty of fruit and vegetables

It is important to include lots of different types of fruit and vegetables in the diet to provide vitamins, minerals, fibre and antioxidant phytochemicals (see Q2.8 and Q2.9). Large portions of vegetables should be served with meals, or salad and fruit should be included as snacks and desserts throughout the day. A minimum of five portions of fruit and vegetables should be included in the diet daily.

Don't eat too many foods that contain a lot of fat

Current fat intakes are higher than the recommended levels. We should aim to reduce fat intakes, on average, from the current level of about 38% to 35% of food energy. Avoiding too many fried foods, choosing lean meat and lower fat dairy foods, and eating cakes, biscuits and chocolates only in moderation should help ensure that fat intakes are within the healthy eating guidelines.

Don't have sugary foods too often

Frequent consumption of sugary foods can increase risk of tooth decay. Sugar-containing foods and drinks can be part of a healthy balanced diet. However, it is advisable to consume these foods as part of a meal rather than constantly throughout the day (see Q1.8).

If you drink alcohol, drink sensibly

Current guidelines on alcohol consumption are that women should consume no more than two to three units a day and men should consume no more than three to four units a day. This is a daily, not a weekly, recommendation, so, for example, it would be unwise to consume the total amount in one go (see Q3.75 and Q3.85).

Q1.7 What is the balance of good health?

Overall, though, it is important to remember that there is no such thing as a good or bad food. Eating is about enjoyment and all foods can be included in a healthy diet, as long as the right balance is achieved. The *National Food Selection Guide: The Balance of Good Health*, developed by the Health Education Authority (1995) and now available from the Food Standards Agency, is a useful pictorial representation of a healthy diet. The guide (Figure 1.2) is divided into five food groups: fruit and vegetables; starchy foods; meat, fish and

The Balance of Good Health

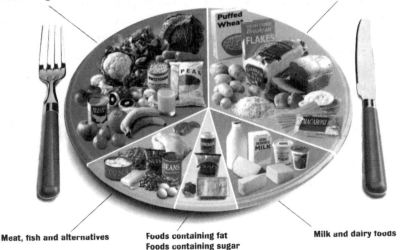

Figure 1.2 The Balance of Good Health. (Reproduced with permission from the British Nutrition Foundation.)

alternatives; milk and dairy foods; and foods containing fat and those containing sugar. The guide is shaped like a dinner plate, which makes it simple to understand and interpret. It can be used to help plan individual meals as well as a balanced diet over a day or more.

Q1.8 What do each of the groups in the 'Balance of Good Health' represent?

The food groups in the 'Balance of Good Health' are as follows.

Bread, other cereals and potatoes

These foods should provide most of our dietary energy, in the form of starch. The amounts that should be consumed will vary with energy needs (see Table 1.1) and appetite (see Q1.6).

Fruit and vegetables

Aim for at least five portions of a wide variety of fruit and vegetables every day to optimise intake of vitamins (especially vitamin C), minerals and fibre, as well as plant constituents (phytochemicals) beneficial to health (see Q2.9).

Meat, fish and alternatives

Two to three portions a day of lean meat, skinless poultry, fish, pulses or nuts should provide an adequate iron intake. Lean meat and reduced fat meat products are the best choices as these are lower in fat. Haem iron, present in meat and fish, is better absorbed than the non-haem iron found in vegetables, pulses and nuts. By including a source of vitamin C with the non-haem iron sources (e.g. citrus or soft fruit) absorption will be enhanced (see Q2.20). This may be an important consideration for vegetarians. Iron-deficiency anaemia is one of the most common deficiencies in the UK, particularly in young children, teenage girls and women of child-bearing age. Promotion of a good intake of iron-containing foods is an important strategy to help prevent this problem (see Q2.6).

Milk and dairy products

Two to three portions a day of milk and dairy products, such as cheese, yoghurt and fromage frais, should provide an adequate calcium intake. The best choices are the lower-fat varieties, of which there is a wide selection available in today's shops and supermarkets. Calcium is important for strong bones. A good intake of calcium, particularly during puberty and early adulthood, in combination with physical activity, can help optimise peak bone mass and delay fractures later in life (see Q2.5).

Foods containing fat and those containing sugar

These foods can be enjoyed, in moderation, as part of a healthy balanced diet. Fatty foods should not, however, be consumed in excess. Sugary foods should, ideally, be consumed with meals, rather than frequently throughout the day (see Q1.6 and Q2.2).

This guide is not applicable to children under 2 years of age, whose fat intakes should not be restricted. This age group should be encouraged to consume a nutrient-dense diet (i.e. a high ratio of nutrients to energy). Between the ages of 2 and 5 years, children should make a gradual change to a more adult diet, and the 'Balance of Good Health' can begin to apply (see Q3.52–3.58).

Q1.9 How does the 'Balance of Good Health' apply to composite meals?

The 'Balance of Good Health' largely depicts single foods, rather than composite meals, but this should not be taken to mean that the latter are unacceptable. For example, a pizza with a thick base and tomatoes, reduced-fat cheese, lean ham and lots of vegetables as a topping would contain all the food groups, in the right proportions for health. Lasagne, with lean minced meat, pasta and a cheese sauce, served with a generous portion of vegetables or salad, is another example of a balanced meal. It does not matter whether the overall diet is composed of composite foods or individual foods, or a mixture of the two; it is more important to ensure that the overall balance of the food groups over a period of, say, one day is in line with the proportions depicted in the 'Balance of Good Health'.

Q1.10 So in terms of health, where are we now?

Fats

Although progress has been made, there is still room for improvement in the UK and elsewhere. According to National Food Survey data for 1999 (MAFF, 2000), the average proportion of food energy derived from total fat and saturated fatty acids was 38.3% and 14.9%, respectively (household consumption). This is in excess of the current recommendations of 35% of food energy from total fat and 11% from saturated fatty acids (see Q1.6 and Q2.3).

Fibre

Intake of fibre (as NSP) in the 1999 household diet was just 11.9 g/person per day. Total fibre intake may be in excess of this but, nevertheless, this falls considerably short of the recommendation of 18 g/day for adults (see Q1.3 and Q2.1).

Fruit and vegetables

There needs to be a focus on the promotion of increased intakes of fruit and vegetables. The Health Survey for England 1994 (Department of Health, 1996a) found that just 14% of men and 21% of women ate fruit more than once a day. The corresponding figures for vegetable consumption were 8% and 13%, respectively. Average consumption was lower among the lower socioeconomic groups. The National Food Survey 1998 (MAFF, 1999) shows that fruit and vegetable consumption over the preceding 10 years was fairly static. There is clearly much work to be done in increasing awareness of the importance of consuming a variety of at least five portions of fruit and vegetables a day. The Government is looking at various initiatives that may help achieve this.

Alcohol

The Health Survey for England in 1996 (Department of Health, 1998b) found that 30% of men were drinking more than 21 units of alcohol per week and 15% of women were drinking more than 14 units of alcohol per week. This is considerably in excess of the original 'Health of the Nation' target to reduce the number of people consuming excess alcohol to 18% of men and 7% of women. The *Our Healthier Nation* report (Department of Health, 1999) recognises that alcohol-related ill-health needs to be tackled, but there are no clear targets set for reducing alcohol consumption (see Q3.75, Q3.85 and Q3.94).

Food Processing

Q1.11 Why is modern food processing considered so important in achieving a
        healthy diet?

Food processing encompasses any action applied to food to render it
safe, edible and more palatable. It can be very traditional, e.g. baking
of flour to make bread, or more modern, e.g. extrusion cooking to
make breakfast cereal. Food processing enables the extension of the
shelf-life of perishable foods and, with the technology available
today, the needs of modern, urban populations can be sustained.
They would not be sustainable without food processing.

Practically all foods undergo some form of food processing before
they are eaten. This may be of a minor nature, e.g. peeling an orange
or boiling some potatoes, or may be more complex, e.g. canning or
sterilisation. Food-processing techniques have meant that there is a
huge diversity of foods available, both in and out of season. It has
also enabled the development of products that meet consumer
demands in terms of health, e.g. salt, sugar, fat and fibre contents can
be manipulated, and foods can be fortified with a range of vitamins
and minerals to enhance their nutritional value or to tackle public
health problems (see Q1.12 and Q3.112).

Q1.12 What is the role of food fortification in achieving a balanced diet?

Fortification can be statutory or voluntary. It involves the addition of
one or more nutrients to a food, over and above the amount that
would normally be present, with the purpose of preventing or
correcting a deficiency of a particular nutrient within the population
as a whole, or within a particular population group. Examples of
fortification are as follows:

- the statutory addition of calcium to all types of flours (other than
  wholemeal) (see Q2.5);
- the statutory addition of vitamins A and D to margarine (see
  Q2.22 and Q3.16);
- the voluntary addition of vitamin A and D to low/reduced fat
  spreads;
- the voluntary addition of vitamins and minerals to breakfast cereals (see Q2.22);

- the voluntary addition of folic acid to breads and breakfast cereals (see Q3.112);
- the voluntary fortification of salt with iodine.

Consumption of fortified foods can make an important contribution to the nutrient intake of some members of the population. It is important to be cautious, however, when considering fortification of a food. Increased folic acid intakes have been shown to be beneficial in preventing neural tube defects in the first 12 weeks of pregnancy (MRC Vitamin Study Group, 1991), and low folate status may be a risk factor for heart disease. There are, therefore, obvious benefits to fortifying foods with folic acid. High intakes of folic acid may not, however, be beneficial in other groups, e.g. high intakes of folic acid could mask vitamin B_{12} deficiency in elderly people or in vegans. It is important to consider the level of a nutrient that will provide maximum benefit to those who need it, without causing adverse effects to other population groups. The recent COMA report on folic acid recommended universal fortification of flour at 240 µg/day per 100 g of food as consumed. This level of fortification was estimated to reduce the risk of neural tube defects by 40%, without resulting in unacceptably high intakes in any group in the population (Department of Health, 2000d).

Q1.13 What are E numbers?

E numbers are used to indicate additives approved for use in foods and that are considered safe throughout the European Community. Additives are listed on food labels either by their chemical name or by their E number.

Additives may be used to enhance the organoleptic qualities of the food, or to prolong the shelf-life and prevent contamination by micro-organisms. The main categories of additives include the following:

- Preservatives which are extremely important in foods because they help to prevent contamination with bacteria, fungi and moulds. Examples of preservatives include vinegar (E260), e.g. in pickled vegetables; nitrates and nitrites (E249–252), e.g. in cured meats; and sulphur dioxide (E220), e.g. in dried apricots.
- Antioxidants which help to prevent fats and oils going rancid. Some are nutrients in their own right, e.g. ascorbic acid (vitamin C) and α-tocopherol (vitamin E) (see Q2.8 and Q4.2).

- Emulsifiers and stabilisers which help to mix oil and water, e.g. foods such as margarine, mayonnaise and ice cream could not exist without the use of emulsifiers. Many emulsifiers are derived from natural products, e.g. lecithin, present in soya beans; guar gum from a plant of the pea family; and alginates from seaweed.
- Colours which are added to foods to enhance natural colour or to replace colour lost in processing, and to ensure uniformity in all products. There are over 40 permitted colours, around half of which are derivatives of natural plant pigments, e.g. those found in green peppers, grape skins or beetroot.
- Flavourings which are added to foods during processing to ensure that the end product tastes good.
- Acidulants which create an acid environment in food. This both contributes to taste and helps to prevent the growth of micro-organisms. The most widely used acidulant is citric acid.
- Intense sweeteners which are used widely in food products as an alternative to sugar. Artificial sweeteners, such as saccharine (400 times sweeter than sugar) and aspartame (200 times sweeter than sugar), are low in calories (energy) and safer for the teeth.

Additives have, over recent years, received a bad press. There have been consumer concerns over safety of additives and suggested links with food intolerance. There are, however, many benefits to food additives as listed above. To be permitted for use in foods there must be evidence of need and the additive must be shown to be safe and beneficial. Furthermore, intolerance to food additives has been shown to be extremely rare, probably affecting just 1 in 10 000 people (see Q4.34). The benefit of adding additives to foods can therefore be judged to far outweigh any possible risk to health.

Nutrition Labelling

Q1.14 How can I get the most out of nutrition labelling?

Legislation governing nutrition labelling requires that a nutrition label must accompany packaged foodstuffs displaying a nutrition claim. This has to be in the formats known as the 'Big 4' or the 'Big 8' (Table 1.8). If, for example, a claim is made relating to the content

Table 1.8 Nutrition labelling formats

Group 1: The Big 4 Declaration

NUTRIENT INFORMATION

Typical values	Per 100g
Energy	kJ/Kcal
Protein	g
Carbohydrates	g
Fat	g

Group 2: The Big 8 Declaration

NUTRIENT INFORMATION

Typical values	Per 100g
Energy	kJ/Kcal
Protein	g
Carbohydrates	g
of which sugars	g
Fat	g
of which saturates	g
Fibre	g
Sodium	g

of sugars, saturates, fibre or sodium, the 'Big 8' must be declared on the label. If no nutrition claim is made, then labelling is voluntary.

There is much confusion among consumers when it comes to interpreting the nutrition label; surveys indicate that many people think that the information is complex and difficult to understand. As a result, the Institute of Grocery Distribution (IGD) conducted research in 1995 that aimed to identify a labelling format for food products that would provide consumers with information to enable them to gain an improved understanding of the nutritional value of foods (Institute of Grocery Distribution, 1998). Their research findings showed that current levels of nutrition understanding among consumers were low and information on the label was perceived as too complicated, frustrating and often illegible. Terms such as carbohydrate, saturates and sodium were not understood and kilojoules were perceived as irrelevant. In 1997, the IGD's voluntary nutrition labelling guidelines were published as a result of this research. These are as follows:

- Fat and calories per serving should be given independently of the main nutrition information table and 'per serving' measures should be stated in household units.
- Guideline daily amounts (GDAs) should be widely promoted by industry. GDAs are predicted daily consumption levels of nutrients based on an average consumer eating a diet that conforms to the current healthy eating recommendations. GDAs are given as 2000 kcal/day – 70 g/day of fat and 20 g/day of saturates – for women, and 2500 kcal/day – 95 g/day fat and 30 g/day of saturates – for men.
- The order of the information on the panel should be changed so that per serving information comes before per 100 g information.
- Saturates were poorly understood by consumers, and it was concluded that it would be inappropriate to highlight saturates on the label at this time.
- Nutritional information should be legible.

Since these guidelines were published, the IGD has been conducting research with consumers to identify whether a salt (or sodium) GDA might be helpful. Also, the Food Standards Agency has announced its intention to consider the need for changes in nutrition labelling.

Q1.15 How useful are health claims on foods?

Any product intended for consumption is defined in law as either a food or a medicine. It cannot be defined as both because different legislation applies. Under food labelling law, medicinal claims cannot be made, i.e. a food cannot be claimed to cure or prevent a specific disease. It is recognised, however, that there is a role for diet in promoting good health and there is also a need to prevent the use of claims that are false, exaggerated or misleading, particularly as the market for functional foods looks set to increase. As a result, the Joint Health Claims Initiative was set up in the UK in June 1997 to establish a code of practice for health claims on foods. This was a joint venture between consumer organisations, enforcement authorities and industry bodies.

A strong consensus emerged in the development of this code that the current legal and enforcement framework governing claims is too permissive in some areas and too restrictive in others. A voluntary code has now been drawn up that adds both rigor and flexibility to the existing system. It was launched formally in December 2000. Information is given on a whole range of issues, including principles and substantiation for making health claims, and labelling and other consumer information. It is hoped that this initiative will help to provide accurate and clear information to consumers about the role of a healthy diet in maintaining good health and treating disease. A recommendation has been made to Ministers to reassess the existing law, to the benefit of the consumer. More information on this initiative is available from Leatherhead Food RA (see Useful addresses).

Functional Foods

Q1.16 What is a functional food?

There is an increasing interest in, and a growing market for, functional foods in the UK today and this is likely to continue into the future (see Q5.6). A functional food may be defined as a food having health-promoting benefits and/or disease-preventing properties over and above its basic nutritional value. Functional foods encompass a broad range of products and can include foods generated around a particular functional ingredient, e.g. stanol-enriched margarine (see Q5.7 and Q5.8), through to staple everyday foods fortified with a nutrient that would not normally be present to any great extent (e.g. folic acid-fortified bread or breakfast cereals). There are four mechanisms, which have been defined below, that could make a food more 'functional':

1. Elimination of a component that has a negative effect, e.g. allergenic or toxic substances.
2. Increased concentration of a component that has a positive effect, e.g. dietary fibre.
3. Addition of a particular ingredient, such as a vitamin, mineral or probiotic culture.
4. Partial replacement of a negative component with a benign or positive component, e.g. a fat substitute.

The potential market for functional foods is enormous, but there is a real need for sound and comprehensive scientific evidence to underpin any health claims made in relation to these foods. Functional foods must be viewed in the context of a healthy diet and lifestyle. They are not a magic solution, or indeed an alternative, for healthy eating. Lifestyle factors such as avoidance of smoking, maintaining a healthy body weight and consumption of a balanced and varied diet are factors that should be given the highest priority in terms of health promotion and disease prevention.

Q1.17 What do the terms probiotic and prebiotic mean?

The healthy human gut contains a large population of micro-organisms, the profile of which can be influenced to some extent by the type of foods consumed. There is currently a growing interest in the use of prebiotics and probiotics, in terms of their influence on colonic microflora and subsequent impact on health. Prebiotics and probiotics can be defined as follows:

- Prebiotics are non-digestible food ingredients that beneficially affect the host by selectively stimulating the growth and/or activity of one or a limited number of types of bacteria in the colon, which can improve host health. Examples of prebiotics include fructo-oligosaccharides (e.g. inulin), raffinose, palatinose, stachyose, xylose, maltose, mannose and lactulose.
- Probiotics are foods that incorporate live micro-organisms. Probiotics have been defined as 'a live microbial feed supplement that beneficially affects the host animal by improving its intestinal microbial balance'. The usual vehicles for probiotics are fermented dairy products, e.g. yoghurt-type products.

A number of health benefits have been ascribed to both prebiotics and probiotics. Evidence of a beneficial effect is, however, at the present time controversial. Some scientific studies do show verifiable evidence of a beneficial effect but other studies are inconclusive. Despite this, there is evidence accumulating to show a health benefit with selected probiotic micro-organisms if they are consumed regularly.

Chapter 2
Nutrients and Health

As explained in Chapter 1, there are no 'good' or 'bad' foods, but an imbalance in the choice of food does exist in the UK and other developed countries. This chapter outlines the role of individual nutrients in the body and describes their importance for health.

Fibre

Q2.1 Why is fibre important?

Dietary fibre (non-starch polysaccharides or NSP) is important for a number of reasons, particularly because it comprises a number of different substances that fall into two distinct categories – soluble fibre and insoluble fibre.

Soluble fibre, as its name suggests, is able to form a gel after consumption, although it passes through the small intestine unabsorbed. This type of fibre is found in fruit (e.g. apples), vegetables, pulses and some grains (especially oats). It is now recognised that the bacteria naturally present in the gut are able to digest soluble fibre, producing a series of short-chain fatty acids: acetic acid, propionic acid and butyric acid. These can be absorbed from the colon into the cells lining the colon, providing an energy source. They can also pass through into the bloodstream. In addition, there is some evidence that propionic acid (absorbed into the bloodstream) can help reduce blood cholesterol levels (see British Nutrition Foundation, 1993), and it has been suggested that butyric acid helps protect the cells lining the colon from precancerous change (German, 1999).

Insoluble fibre is found in grains and fibrous vegetables. It has a bulking effect on faeces and so decreases transit time through the gut. Current advice is to aim to eat a variety of fibre sources on a regular basis. Average daily fibre intake in Britain is only 12 g/day, whereas the dietary reference value (DRV) is 18 g/day for adults. Those on a low-fibre intake should increase their consumption gradually (Department of Health, 1991).

Resistant starch does not fall within the category of NSP, but it is also thought to contribute to bacterial fermentation. It is provided, in varying amounts, by a number of starchy foods.

Sugar

Q2.2 Should we be concerned about sugar intake?

Sugar is a generic name for a range of substances of similar structure, e.g. sucrose (table sugar), fructose (found in fruit), lactose (found in milk) and glucose. All of these sugars provide 4 kcal/g (17 kJ/g) of energy. Although sugars can contribute towards over-consumption of energy in an imbalanced diet, the main concern relates to oral health. In this context, it is the frequency of sugar consumption, rather than the actual amount eaten, that is associated with dental caries risk.

Current advice is to restrict consumption of sugar-rich foods and drinks to four or five occasions per day, ideally keeping to meal times. This is because, each time sugar is eaten, the pH at the tooth surface falls as bacteria present in dental plaque ferment the sugar, producing acid. It is this acid that attacks dental enamel. To prevent caries, it is important to restrict the number of times that teeth are exposed to these acidic conditions. Consequently, eating sugary foods and drinks in one go, rather than over a protracted period between meals, makes sense. There is less concern about sugars naturally present in fruit and milk, and there is no evidence that these foods contribute to dental decay if eaten normally. In the case of milk, this may be the result of protective factors in the milk. Indeed, cheese (e.g. Cheddar) is now recognised to be capable of offsetting harmful effects of sugar, if eaten at the same meal as sugar-rich foods (see British Nutrition Foundation, 1999b).

Fat

Q2.3 Why do we need to consider our intake of fat?

The dietary reference value (DRV) for fat intake in Britain is 35% of energy intake (see Q1.6). The actual consumption of fat has fallen considerably over the last 20 years, with household consumption figures showing a drop from 104 g/day per person in the early 1980s to 72 g/day per person in 1999 (MAFF, 2000). However, the contribution of fat to energy intake remains above the recommended value at 38.3% of food energy, according to the latest statistics from the National Food Survey (contribution of household food in the UK). This is because our intake of energy has fallen in parallel, i.e. the choice of lower-fat foods has not been accompanied by an increased consumption of starchy foods. Despite this fall in energy intake, the prevalence of obesity has been steadily rising; this is thought to result from the fact that we have, concurrently, become less physically active (see Q4.5–4.12).

A high intake of fat is considered a health risk for a number of reasons. It is associated with an increased risk of heart disease and some cancers. It is also more likely to result in excessive energy consumption because high-fat foods are energy dense and usually very palatable. In particular, it is important to consider intake of the various types of fatty acids.

Q2.4 What are the different types of fatty acid and what are the health implications?

Fatty acids are the building blocks from which other fats (lipids) in the body are made. In food, fat is usually in the form of triacylglycerols (triglycerides). These are also the main storage form of fat in the body and usually consist of three different fatty acids attached to a backbone of glycerol (Figure 2.1). In most natural fats and oils, specific fatty acids tend to be located at particular positions on the backbone, although at least one of the fatty acids is usually selected randomly. The physical properties of fats and oils are influenced largely by the nature of their constituent fatty acids.

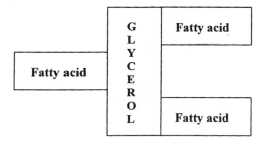

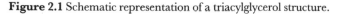

Figure 2.1 Schematic representation of a triacylglycerol structure.

All fatty acids are made up of a string of carbon atoms, to which are attached hydrogen atoms, forming a hydrocarbon chain. Fatty acids can be saturated or unsaturated.

Saturated

When each of the carbon atoms (except the two at the ends of the chain) is bonded to two hydrogen atoms, the fatty acid is said to be saturated – all the bonding capacity of the carbons is saturated with hydrogen.

Unsaturated

When each of two adjacent carbon atoms in the chain (except the two at the ends of the chain) is bonded to only one hydrogen, a rigid link (double bond) exists between the pair of carbons and the fatty acid is said to be unsaturated. If the chain contains only one rigid link, it is said to be monounsaturated. If the fatty acid has two or more rigid links, it is known as a polyunsaturated fatty acid. There are two distinct families of polyunsaturated fatty acids, n-6 and n-3. These are also sometimes known as omega-6 (ω-6) and omega-3 (ω-3).

The hydrogen atoms on either side of a double bond may be on the same side of the unsaturated fatty acid molecule, in which case the fatty acid is said to have a *cis* configuration, or on opposite sides giving the *trans* configuration. Fatty acids with one or more *cis* double bonds are more abundant in nature than those with one or more *trans* double bonds. Most of the *trans*-fatty acids we consume are produced during the hydrogenation (hardening) process that converts vegetable oils into solid fats. However, they are also naturally present in milk and milk products as a direct result of the fermentation process that takes place in the cow's gastrointestinal tract.

It is important to consider not only the total amount of fat in the diet, but also the proportions of different fatty acids. Dietary recommendations for intake of fatty acids are given in the report of the Committee on Medical Aspects of Food Policy (COMA) on Nutritional Aspects of Cardiovascular Disease (Department of Health, 1994b). This report recommended that intakes of saturated fatty acids (SFAs) should be reduced to no more than about 10% of food energy. This is slightly lower than the recommendation of 11% of food energy from SFAs, which was made in the report on dietary reference values (Department of Health, 1991). Average intakes of *trans*-fatty acids should not increase.

No specific recommendations have been made for monounsaturated fatty acids (MUFAs). Rich sources of monounsaturated fatty acids include olive oil and the far more economical rapeseed oil. These fatty acids are often associated with the Mediterranean diet and are thought to be beneficial to health, in moderation, particularly if they replace saturated fatty acids and provided that total fat intake remains within the recommended guidelines. This class of fatty acid is also found in moderate amounts in meat and in dairy products.

Average intakes of *n*-6 polyunsaturated fatty acids (PUFAs) need not increase above current levels and intakes of very-long-chain *n*-3 PUFAs should double from 0.1 g/day to 0.2 g/day (Department of Health, 1994b).

One of the *n*-6 fatty acids, linoleic acid, is essential in the diet because it cannot be made in the body. This fatty acid is also recognised to help reduce blood cholesterol levels, and so its intake via foods has been encouraged (see Q3.93 and Q4.2). As a result, over recent decades, the ratio of *n*-6:*n*-3 fatty acids in the UK diet has increased. This is a result of increasing use of vegetable oils rich in *n*-6 (e.g. sunflower oil) in cooking, baked and other manufactured foods, and in margarines and spreads, coupled with a reduction in oil-rich fish intake. Oil-rich fish are the richest source of the very-long-chain *n*-3 fatty acids known as eicosapentaenoic acid (EPA) and docosahexaenoic acid (DHA). These fatty acids have very important functions in the body, e.g. they are essential structural components in the brain and also beneficially influence blood lipids. Their impact is on blood triglycerides rather than cholesterol, which is not substantially changed by 'fish-oil' fatty acids (see Q4.2).

Although EPA and DHA (fish-oil fatty acids) are important, they can be made from the shorter-chain essential *n*-3 fatty acid, α-linolenic acid, present in some vegetable and seed oils. For those readers interested in finding out more about *n*-3 fatty acids, a Briefing Paper on the subject is available from the British Nutrition Foundation (British Nutrition Foundation, 1999c).

It is often not recognised that most foods provide a mixture of fatty acid types, although one sort often predominates. No single source of fat is wholly saturated or wholly polyunsaturated (Table 2.1).

Table 2.1 Typical fatty acid composition of some foods

	g/100 g food	Fatty acids (% of fat by weight)[a]		
		Saturated	Monounsaturated	Polyunsaturated
Butter	82.2	72	25	3
Margarine, soft	80.0	35	47	18
Margarine, polyunsaturated	68.5	25	23	52
Rapeseed oil	99.9	7	62	31
Sunflower oil	99.9	13	21	66
Milk, whole cows'	4.0	71	26	3
Eggs	11.2	35	47	18
Cheese, Cheddar	32.7	71	26	3
Beef, mince	15.7	51	47	2
Pork, chops	15.7	38	44	18
Biscuits, chocolate chip	22.9	49	39	12
Potato crisps	11.0	68	30	2
Peanuts	46.0	20	50	30

[a]Figures calculated for *cis*-fatty acids; *trans* have not been included (MAFF, 1998a).

Other Nutrients and Phytochemicals

Q2.5 Why are there concerns about calcium intake?

Calcium has a primary structural role in bones and teeth (see Q3.98). It is also essential for communication between cells and within cells. Milk and milk products are major providers of calcium. Bread also contributes significantly to calcium intake as a consequence of the statutory fortification of flour. Other sources include pulses, green vegetables and, if eaten regularly, dried fruit, nuts and seeds and the soft bones found in tinned fish (see Q1.8 and Q3.67). Bran-enriched foods, as opposed to wholemeal or wholegrain, can block absorption of calcium because of their high phytate content.

Q2.6 Why are there concerns about iron intake?

Iron is a component of haemoglobin, myoglobin and many other enzymes, e.g. cytochrome P450 (important in drug metabolism). Deficiency causes defective red cell synthesis and hence anaemia. Adverse effects on work capacity, intellectual performance and behaviour can occur.

Meat (particularly red meat) and meat products are a rich source of well-absorbed iron (haem iron) (see Q1.8 and Q3.66). Other important sources of iron are cereal products, particularly bread and breakfast cereals, but also other products made from fortified flour and vegetables. (Iron is also found in eggs, beans, e.g. baked beans and lentils, potatoes and dried fruit.) To aid iron absorption from plant sources, a food or drink that contains vitamin C (e.g. fresh orange juice) should be consumed at the same meal as the iron-containing food (see Q2.20). Tea and phytate-rich cereal products (e.g. bran-enriched) should not be consumed with iron because they inhibit iron absorption.

Q2.7 Which foods are important for protein?

The amount of protein in different foods varies, but the main sources include meat, poultry, fish, cheese, milk, eggs, cereals, nuts and pulses. In the average UK diet, animal sources of protein contribute about two-thirds to total intake. Protein from animal sources tends to have a higher biological value than protein from plant sources; this means that they contain more of the indispensable (essential) amino acids required by humans.

For those people following a vegan diet, it is important to include a variety of plant protein sources. This will help ensure that an appropriate amino acid mix is consumed, because the different foods will complement each other. In particular, foods such as cereals, nuts, peas, beans and lentils are useful sources of protein for a vegan (see Q1.8).

Q2.8 What are antioxidant nutrients?

Antioxidant vitamins include vitamins C and E and pro-vitamin A carotenoids. The minerals selenium, manganese, zinc and copper are also important in this respect because they can be incorporated into enzymes with antioxidant properties, which have key functions in the body. These nutrients are thought to help prevent oxidation reactions in the body, which can lead to cellular damage. Ultimately, these nutrients may play a role in helping to prevent chronic diseases such as cancer and heart disease. More research is needed in this area, but current advice should be to include a variety of fruit and vegetables in the diet, which are good sources of some of these nutrients (see Q1.6, Q5.11). Specific sources of these nutrients can be found later in this section.

Q2.9 What are phytochemicals?

Phytochemicals is a term used to encompass substances found in plants (see Q4.2). These include not only nutrients such as vitamin C and β-carotene, but also other substances that may have a beneficial effect on health, e.g. flavonoids (see Q5.9).

Q2.10 Why do we need vitamin A?

Vitamin A is needed for growth and normal development, maintenance and repair of tissues, maintenance of immune function, normal and night vision. It is found in the British diet in two forms:

1. Retinol (pre-formed vitamin A): found in meat and meat products, liver, kidney, milk and milk products derived from whole milk, margarine (fish liver oils).
2. Carotenoids (pro-vitamin A, e.g. β-carotene): found in all vegetables, especially carrots, and red and orange fruit (e.g. tomatoes). (Not all carotenoids are precursors for vitamin A – see Q5.11.)

Q2.11 Why do we need carotenoids such as β-carotene?

There are many carotenoids found in fruit and vegetables. Some carotenoids, e.g. β-carotene, which is the most commonly occurring carotenoid, can be converted into retinol in the body; 6 mg of β-carotene is equivalent to 1 mg of retinol. β-Carotene also has antioxidant properties in its own right (see Q2.8 and Q4.3).

Q2.12 Why do we need thiamin?

Thiamin is involved in the metabolism of fat, carbohydrate and alcohol. All cereals, especially breads and breakfast cereals, and potatoes are significant sources of this vitamin in the British diet. Smaller quantities are provided by a wide range of foods, including meat and meat products, milk and milk products, and vegetables.

Q2.13 Why do we need riboflavin?

Riboflavin is required for oxidative processes and there are a number of enzymes that are flavin dependent. Riboflavin is found in milk and milk products and fortified breakfast cereals, which are the main sources in the British diet. Meat and meat products provide smaller quantities.

Q2.14 Why do we need niacin?

Niacin (nicotinamide and nicotinic acid) is the reactive part of the coenzymes NAD and NADP, and so is very important in intermediary metabolism (e.g. energy production). Niacin requirement is related to energy metabolism. Meat and meat products, bread, fortified breakfast cereals, potatoes, milk and milk products are the main sources of niacin in the British diet (it is also provided by fish).

Q2.15 Why do we need vitamin B_6?

Vitamin B_6, as pyridoxal phosphate, is a cofactor for a large number of enzymes associated with amino acid metabolism. It is widely distributed in foods. Particular sources are potatoes and breakfast cereals (see Q3.77 and Q5.4).

Q2.16 Why do we need vitamin B_{12}?

Vitamin B_{12} is involved in the recycling of folate coenzymes and is needed for nerve myelination. Vitamin B_{12} is found naturally only in foods of animal origin – meat and its products, especially liver, and milk and its products make the major contribution. It is also present in eggs and fish, and is added to fortified breakfast cereals.

Q2.17 Why do we need folate (folic acid)?

Folic acid is a synthetic form of the B vitamin folate. The vitamin is involved in a number of single-carbon transfer reactions, especially in the synthesis of purines, pyrimidines, glycine and methionine. Therefore, deficiency affects blood cell development and growth. Folates are found in: green leafy vegetables (raw or lightly boiled), especially sprouts and spinach; green beans and peas; potatoes; fruit, especially oranges; Bovril and yeast extract; and milk and milk products. Folic acid is added to a number of products these days, especially some breakfast cereals and bread (see Q1.12). Liver is also a good source but should not be consumed by pregnant women or women hoping to conceive, because of the risk of damage to the fetus as a result of excess vitamin A intake. It is now recognised that folic acid can help prevent the occurrence of neural tube defects. All women of child-bearing age embarking on a pregnancy should be encouraged to take a 400 µg/day supplement and to continue this for the first 12 weeks of pregnancy (see Q3.2). There is growing interest in the relationship between folate status and risk of coronary heart disease, but it is yet to be shown that supplements can reduce risk (Department of Health, 2000d; Hughes and Buttriss, 2000).

Q2.18 Why do we need pantothenic acid?

Pantothenic acid is needed for the release of energy from fats, carbohydrates, proteins and alcohol. Experimental deficiency has been found to result in fatigue, headaches, dizziness, muscle weakness and gastrointestinal problems. There is no evidence of deficiency in humans, except in experimental situations. Pantothenic acid is widely distributed in foods, in particular in animal products, wholegrains and legumes.

Q2.19 Why do we need biotin?

Biotin deficiency is rare in humans and has occurred only as a result of bizarre dietary practices or in long-term parenteral nutrition. Deficiency results in scaly dermatitis and hair loss. This vitamin is widely distributed in foods and is synthesised by intestinal micro-organisms.

Q2.20 Why do we need vitamin C?

Vitamin C prevents scurvy and aids wound healing. It also assists in the absorption of non-haem iron and is an important antioxidant (see Q2.6 and Q2.8). However, it can also act as a pro-oxidant in the presence of certain metal ions and oxygen. The richest sources in the British diet are citrus fruit, fruit juices and soft fruit. Other sources include green vegetables, other fruit, peppers and potatoes, especially new potatoes (see Q4.17).

Q2.21 Why do we need vitamin E?

Vitamin E is the major lipid-soluble antioxidant in membranes and hence can be seen as offering protection against free radical damage. Immune function is influenced by vitamin E. Vegetable oils, margarine, wholegrain cereals, eggs, vegetables (especially dark-green leafy types) and nuts provide most of the vitamin E in the British diet.

Q2.22 Why do we need vitamin D?

In its active form, 1,25-dihydroxy-vitamin D (1,25-$(OH)_2$D), vitamin D is involved in calcium homoeostasis. As well as helping to control plasma calcium levels, it may also have a direct effect on bone (see Q3.98). Exposure of skin to sunlight results in the manufacture of vitamin D, but there are few dietary sources of vitamin D. Oil-rich fish such as herring, pilchards, sardines and tuna, meat, eggs, and fortified foods including margarine, some yoghurts, evaporated milk and breakfast cereals are the main sources in the British diet (see Q3.16, Q3.98).

Q2.23 Why do we need vitamin K?

Vitamin K is needed for the synthesis of procoagulant factors. It may also be important for a strong skeleton (see Q3.98). Green leafy vegetables are the richest source in the British diet. It is also found in other vegetables, fruit, dairy produce, vegetable oils, cereals and meat. (See Buttriss et al., 2000 for a review of vitamin K.)

Q2.24 Why do we need selenium?

Selenium is an integral part of the enzyme glutathione peroxidase, which is one of the enzymes that protects against oxidative damage. Another selenoprotein is involved in thyroid hormone synthesis. Cereals, meat and fish contribute the bulk of the selenium in the British diet. Brazil nuts can be particularly rich, although the amount present is very variable. The amount present in cereals (and other plants) is determined by the soil type. The role of selenium in health is the subject of a recent British Nutrition Foundation Briefing Paper (British Nutrition Foundation, 2001a).

Q2.25 Why do we need magnesium?

Magnesium is involved in skeletal development (intimately involved in calcium metabolism) and in the maintenance of electrical potential in nerve and muscle membranes. It acts as a cofactor for enzymes involved in energy utilisation, in the replication of DNA and the synthesis of RNA. Main sources are cereals, cereal products, e.g. bread (particularly wholegrain/wholemeal), and green vegetables. Some magnesium is also found in milk and a small amount is contributed by meat and potatoes. Nuts and seeds are also quite rich in magnesium.

Q2.26 Why do we need phosphorus?

Along with calcium, phosphorus is a constituent of the substance, hydroxyapatite, that gives bones their rigidity. It is also a constituent of all the major classes of biochemical compounds – the energy that drives most metabolic processes is derived from the phosphate bond in ATP. Phosphorus in the form of phosphate is present in all foods and is also present in many food additives. Particular sources are milk and milk products, bread and meat products (including poultry).

Q2.27 Why do we need potassium?

Potassium is principally an intracellular cation and, like sodium, is involved in acid/base regulation, generation of transmembrane concentration gradients, and electrical conductivity in nerves and muscles. It is particularly abundant in vegetables, potatoes, fruit (especially bananas) and juices. It is also found in bread, fish, nuts and seeds. Meat and milk also contribute to intake but these foods, particularly processed meat products and cheese, also provide some sodium, thus reducing the potassium:sodium ratio.

Q2.28 Why do we need sodium and why are there concerns about excessive intakes?

Sodium is the principal cation in extracellular fluid (ECF) and is involved in ECF volume and osmotic pressure maintenance, acid/base balance, electrical conductivity in muscles and nerves, and the generation of transmembrane concentration gradients involved in uptake of nutrients by cells. Traditionally, sodium (in the form of sodium chloride, salt) has been used as a preservative and flavour enhancer. The main sources are processed foods: bread and cereal products, breakfast cereals; meat products; pickles; canned vegetables; tinned and packet sauces and soups, and savoury snack foods. Spreading fats and cheese also make a relatively small contribution to intake. An important source for some people is salt added at the table and during cooking.

There is concern about excessive intakes in relation to high blood pressure, and some individuals may be particularly salt sensitive. It is important to note, however, that other factors are also important in affecting blood pressure, notably obesity and alcohol intake (see Q4.2). Reducing salt intake, however, may be one appropriate dietary strategy in those who are hypertensive. Other dietary factors include eating plenty of fruit and vegetables (rich in potassium) and low-fat dairy products (rich in calcium). (For further information see Q1.8, Q2.26 and Q4.2.)

Q2.29 Why do we need zinc?

Zinc is involved in the major metabolic pathways contributing to the metabolism of proteins, carbohydrates, energy, nucleic acids and lipids. Hence, inadequate intakes are reflected in growth retardation, and in adverse effects on tissues with rapid turnover, e.g. skin and the intestinal mucosa, and the immune system. Significant sources in the British diet include meat, meat products, milk and its products, and bread and cereal products (especially wholemeal varieties). Other sources include eggs, beans and lentils, nuts, sweetcorn and rice. Absorption of minerals such as zinc is relatively poor from phytate-rich cereals, such as unleavened bread.

Q2.30 Why do we need copper?

Copper is a component of a number of enzymes including cytochrome oxidase, superoxide dismutase, and enzymes involved in the synthesis of neuroactive peptides. Although shellfish and liver are particularly rich in copper, the main sources in the British diet are meat, bread and other cereal products, and vegetables. Drinking water can make an important contribution, particularly when the water is supplied via copper piping.

Q2.31 Why do we need iodine?

Iodine forms part of the hormones thyroxine and triiodothyronine, which help control metabolic rate, cellular metabolism and integrity of connective tissue. Thyroid hormone synthesis is also reliant on selenium (see Q 2.24). In the first 3 months of gestation, iodine is needed for the development of the nervous system. Fish and sea vegetables (e.g. kelp) are rich sources, but milk and milk products are a major source of iodine in the UK. Beer can also be a significant source, as can meat products. The use of iodised table salt, although not common in the UK, is beneficial in areas where iodine deficiency is common.

Q2.32 Why do we need manganese?

Manganese is a component of a number of enzymes and is necessary for the activation of others. Tea is a major source. Other sources include wholegrain cereals, bread, vegetables, nuts and seeds.

Q2.33 Why do we need molybdenum?

Molybdenum is essential for the functioning of a number of enzymes involved in the metabolism of DNA and sulphites. Molybdenum is widely distributed, but is found particularly in vegetables, bread and other cereals. Other sources include milk and milk products, eggs and pulses.

Q2.34 Why do we need chromium?

Chromium seems to be necessary for potentiating the action of insulin. It may also be involved in lipoprotein metabolism, in gene expression and in maintaining the structure of nucleic acids. Foods rich in chromium include brewer's yeast, meat products, cheese, wholegrains and condiments (and legumes and nuts). Cereals and meat are among the largest contributors to intake.

Q2.35 Why do we need chloride?

Chloride is the major extracellular and intracellular counter to sodium and potassium. Dietary sources include salt (sodium chloride) and foods containing it (see sodium), such as bread, meat products and dairy products (see Q2.28).

Q2.36 Why do we need fluoride?

Fluoride (fluorine) forms calcium fluoroapatite in teeth and bone. It protects against tooth decay and may have a role in bone mineralisation. Significant sources in the British diet include tea (probably via the water). It is also provided by fish and, in some areas, drinking water contains added fluoride.

Q2.37 Supplements versus foods?

Most healthy people are able to meet their requirements for vitamins and minerals by eating a varied balanced diet which includes lean meat, dairy products and lots of starchy foods, fruit and vegetables. However, some groups may have high requirements and so may need to take vitamin or mineral supplements:

- Infants and children are recommended to take supplement drops containing vitamins A, C and D from 6 months until 2 years of age and preferably until the age of 5 years (see Q3.31 and Q3.51).
- Pregnant women and breast-feeding mothers may require vitamin D supplements to achieve intakes of 10 µg/day (see Q3.16).
- Any woman planning a baby (or who might become pregnant) and pregnant women up to 12 weeks after conception should take a folic acid supplement of 400 µg/day to reduce the risk of neural tube defects in their babies (see Table 1.2).
- Women with high menstrual losses and those with iron-deficiency anaemia may need iron supplements (see Table 1.3 and Q2.6).
- Elderly or house-bound people, and those who cover up most of their skin, may need a vitamin D supplement of 10 µg/day (see Q3.16, Q3.111 and Q3.113).
- People recovering from illness may have low stores of a number of micronutrients and may benefit from a low-dose multi-vitamin/mineral supplement during their convalescence. There is also growing concern about the poor nutritional status of many people entering hospital, particularly those with chronic disease.

These days, many people take low-dose vitamin and mineral supplements from time to time. However, some vitamins and minerals are toxic at high levels of intake, so it is important to ensure that the manufacturer's guidelines are followed carefully. Some high doses of vitamin supplements are not recommended for certain groups of people:

- High-dose vitamin A supplements are not recommended for pregnant women or those who might become pregnant (see Q3.1).
- A recent Government report on cancer (Department of Health, 1998c) cautions against taking β-carotene supplements as a means of protecting against cancer (in several recent trials, the incidence of cancer actually increased in high-risk individuals taking such supplements) (see Q4.3).

If a vitamin or mineral supplement is taken, this should never be a substitute for a varied balanced diet and the manufacturer's guidelines should not be exceeded.

Chapter 3
Nutrition Through Life

Nutritional needs vary throughout a person's life, although the general principles of a well-balanced diet remain. This chapter outlines the differing needs and health concerns associated with the diets of various groups, including pregnant women, infants, school-children, adolescents and older people.

Nutrition and Preconception

Q3.1 What are the important issues to consider?

The health and nutritional status of women immediately before conception and during the first 3 months of pregnancy is important because this is the time when the growing baby is most susceptible to environmental influences, including dietary imbalances. As many women are unaware of their pregnancy in the early weeks, this only serves to emphasise the importance of increasing awareness of the benefits of good nutrition among women of child-bearing age, which should build on the information provided through health education programmes in schools.

Women should be encouraged to prepare for pregnancy by reducing their alcohol intake (see Q3.6), giving up smoking (see Q3.7) and making adjustments to their diet. In particular, they should be encouraged to take folic acid supplements (see below). Existence of both underweight and overweight are best corrected before conception. Attempts to slim while pregnant may harm the fetus. Low body weight can reduce fertility and overweight women carry an increased risk of complications in late pregnancy, including gestational diabetes and raised blood pressure.

Women who might become pregnant (or are already pregnant) are advised not to consume supplements containing vitamin A (unless specifically advised by their doctor) or to eat liver or liver pâté. This is because, on occasions, these foods can contain very high concentrations of vitamin A (13–40 mg/100 g), and vitamin A in high doses is known to cause congenital malformations. For other dietary sources of vitamin A, see Q2.10.

Entering pregnancy well nourished is important and this is best achieved by eating a varied diet that meets energy requirements (see Table 1.1). Diet before pregnancy and between pregnancies can be as important as diet during pregnancy. In particular, it is important to ensure that intakes of iron, calcium, folate and essential fatty acids are adequate (see Table 1.3 and Q1.2, Q3.78). Particular concern exists about the nutritional status of pregnant adolescent girls (see Q3.15 and Q3.4)

Q3.2 Why are folic acid supplements recommended?

Maternal folate status is now recognised as being important in the avoidance of neural tube defects (NTDs), e.g. spina bifida. For this reason, a folic acid supplement (400 µg/day) is recommended for all women of child-bearing age embarking on a pregnancy (MRC Vitamin Study Group, 1991). Folic acid is the synthetic form of the vitamin folate. This supplement should be taken before conception and continued until week 12 of pregnancy. A larger supplement (4 mg/day) is recommended for women who have already had an NTD pregnancy, to help prevent recurrence. It is particularly important that this group of women should receive advice on folic acid intake. In addition, it is recommended that all women of child-bearing age eat more folate-rich foods (e.g. vegetables) and foods fortified with folic acid (e.g. certain breads and breakfast cereals). (See Q2.17 for other dietary sources of folic acid. This advice has recently been reaffirmed by the Government's advisory committee, COMA (Department of Health, 2000d). The Committee also recommended consideration of a folic acid fortification policy for flour in the UK. A public consultation on this proposal was conducted in late 2000.)

If women who have not been taking a supplement find that they are pregnant, they should start to take supplements immediately and continue until they are 12 weeks' pregnant. This advice supersedes that presented in the COMA DRVs report published in 1991.

Q3.3 What about other supplements?

Apart from folic acid, other vitamin and mineral supplements will normally not be necessary. However, if there is any doubt about the adequacy of a woman's diet, a low-dose multi-vitamin and mineral supplement can be a safeguard. High-dose supplements (greatly in excess of the DRVs) are probably best avoided in women wishing to conceive, especially if there is a chance that they contain vitamin A (see above).

Nutrition and Pregnancy

Q3.4 What aspects of diet are particularly important during pregnancy?

Several studies have suggested that a low birthweight for gestational age, an indicator of poor fetal growth, may increase the risk of degenerative diseases in adult life (Barker, 1992). Although a range of genetic and environmental factors can influence birthweight, an adequate energy and micronutrient intake throughout pregnancy is essential to ensure a healthy environment for fetal growth and development.

The need for some nutrients increases during pregnancy, but the increase in requirement for dietary energy is small in most women, particularly early on in pregnancy (Table 3.1).

As a result of the risks associated with excessive intakes of vitamin A, the Department of Health advises that pregnant women should avoid liver and liver-containing products, such as pâté (see above and see also Q3.1).

Adequate attention to food hygiene is particularly important for pregnant women (see Q5.16). In addition, foods that have been linked with the bacteria *Listeria monocytogenes* should be avoided (e.g. pâtés and mould-ripened soft cheeses, e.g. Brie and Camembert) (see Q3.19).

During pregnancy, additional requirements for a number of nutrients (e.g. calcium) are catered for by an increase in absorption. This means that, provided the woman's intake is in line with recommendations, an increase in dietary supply will not be necessary. An exception to this would be teenage girls who become pregnant, because they are still developing their own skeleton. The RNI for calcium for teenage girls is 800 mg/day rather than 700 mg for older

Table 3.1 Increases in nutrient needs during pregnancy

	Non-pregnant (age 19–50 years)	Pregnant
Energy (kcal)	1940	+200[a]
Protein (g)	45	+6
Thiamin (mg)	0.8	+0.1[a]
Riboflavin (mg)	1.1	+0.3
Niacin (mg)	13.0	No increment
Vitamin B12 (µg)	1.5	No increment
Folate (µg)	200	+100[b]
Vitamin C (mg)	40	+10
Vitamin A (µg)	600	+100
Vitamin D (µg)	No RNI	10
Calcium (mg)	700	No increment
Phosphorus (mg)	550	No increment
Magnesium (mg)	270	No increment
Zinc (mg)	7.0	No increment
Copper (mg)	1.2	No increment
Selenium (µg)	6.0	No increment
Iron (mg)	14.8	No increment

[a]Last trimester only
[b]This recommendation was published before recommendations concerning folic acid supplementation during pregnancy. Women are now advised to take a daily 400µg supplement until week 12 of pregnancy in addition to their normal dietary intake (typically about 200 µg).

women. A similar situation exists for iron: more iron is required during pregnancy, to supply the growing fetus, placenta and increased numbers of maternal red blood cells. However, provided a woman enters pregnancy with adequate iron stores, these stores will be mobilised. Iron absorption will also be increased. In addition, there will be a saving as a result of cessation of menstrual losses. Nevertheless, a large proportion (perhaps as many as 50%) of women of child-bearing age have no iron stores, and so this puts them at increased risk of anaemia should they become pregnant. Ideally, poor iron status should be tackled before pregnancy. Guidelines on expected iron levels for non-pregnant women are 12 g/dl or above for haemoglobin and 12 µg/dl or above for serum ferritin. For pregnant women, the respective figures are 11 g/dl and 12 µg/dl. For women first tested late in pregnancy, haemoglobin levels below

10 g/dl, in association with a mean cell volume (MCV) of 82 fl or less, or a progressive fall in MCV, may indicate the need for dietary intervention and/or supplementation, but this is a complex and highly controversial area.

Q3.5 What is considered a normal weight gain (and energy intake)?

For most women in the UK, the additional energy requirements imposed by pregnancy are quite small and only really apply to the last trimester, when an average of an extra 200 kcal/day is needed. Women who do not reduce their activity levels or are underweight when they conceive may need a little more. On the other hand, some women will need no energy increment because they reduce their physical activity levels substantially.

In the UK, average weight gain in pregnancy is 12.5 kg. The National Academy of Sciences (USA) (1990) has recommended the weight gains shown in Table 3.2.

These recommendations take into account the finding that low gestational weight gain is an important determinant of poor fetal growth and associated with an increased risk of intrauterine growth retardation. For women with a normal pre-pregnancy body mass index, a target weight gain of 0.4 kg/week during the second and third trimester is recommended. For underweight women, the recommendation is 0.5 kg/week and for overweight women 0.3 kg/week. Average weekly weight gain of more than 0.5 kg is considered to be too fast.

Table 3.2 Recommended weight gain during pregnancy

Pre-pregnancy body mass index (BMI)	Recommended gain over the course of the pregnancy (kg)
< 19.8 (underweight)	12.5–18.0
19.8–26.0 (normal weight)	11.5–16.0
26.0–29.0 (overweight)	7.0–11.5

Q3.6 What about alcohol?

Alcohol has been shown to affect ova adversely by affecting the rate of conception and the viability of conception (Crawley, 1993). An intake of 30–40 g/day (4–5 units) has been associated with fetal alcohol syndrome (Abel, 1998). Women who are pregnant, or attempting to conceive, should avoid alcoholic drinks or reduce intake to a minimum. Particular attention should be paid to the folate status of women who are unable to comply with this advice because folate absorption and utilisation are compromised by alcohol (see Q3.85).

Q3.7 What about smoking?

Women should be discouraged from smoking before and during pregnancy, because it is associated with decreased fertility and lower birthweight (Forster et al., 1999). If women are unable to comply with this advice, special attention should be paid to their overall nutrient intake, especially that of vitamin C, in order to help counteract the harmful effects of smoking on the fetus.

Q3.8 What about caffeine?

Claims that consumption of caffeinated beverages is associated with reduced fertility and defects in fetal development have not been substantiated. Whilst moderate intakes (up to four or five cups of instant coffee a day) are unlikely to be harmful for most pregnant women, those at high risk of miscarriage should reduce their intake to one or two cups per day. Cola and tea also contain caffeine and their consumption should be taken into account.

Q3.9 Are there any particular recommendations for women with a history of allergic disease?

Babies whose parents have a history of allergic disease are more likely to go on to develop allergy themselves. It has been suggested that sensitisation to foreign proteins that cross the placenta (or reach the infant via breast milk) may occur in such babies. On the other hand, exposure to a range of potential allergens, via the placenta or via breast milk, during fetal life and infancy enables the baby to develop normal tolerance to the many foreign proteins in the environment. On balance, the benefits of the mother avoiding specific foods during pregnancy and lactation has not been proved and, indeed, this may prevent establishment of a normal immune response to these proteins. As a result of the risks to the baby associated with restrictive diets, which may effectively limit supply of essential nutrients, avoidance of foods known to cause allergy (e.g. milk and milk products, or egg) should be practised only where the baby is seen to be at a severe risk as a result of a strong family history. A British Nutrition Foundation Task Force Report covering this topic is due to be published in late 2001 and a Briefing Paper is now available (British Nutrition Foundation 2000).

Q3.10 What is the advice regarding avoidance of peanut allergy?

Allergy to peanuts seems to be on the increase and is a cause for concern because its effects can be very serious. Allergy to peanut protein can cause anaphylaxis. In a recent review (MAFF, 1998b), it was concluded that the relationship between peanut consumption by pregnant (and breast-feeding) women and the incidence of peanut allergy in their offspring was inconclusive. The latest advice recommends that pregnant women who are atopic (or whose husband or any sibling of the unborn child has an atopic disease) may wish to avoid eating peanuts and peanut products during pregnancy (Department of Health 1998). The same advice applies during lactation. This advice does not apply in the absence of atopy. (See Q3.28 for further information.) A fact sheet on this subject is available on the British Nutrition Foundation's website (www.nutrition.org.uk). (Also see British Nutrition Foundation 2000).

Q3.11 Some women experience constipation or haemorrhoids when they are pregnant. Can diet help?

These conditions are common during pregnancy. Practical advice to pregnant women should be to increase intake of fibre, by increasing intake of complex (starchy) carbohydrate, particularly wholegrain cereals and breads (see Q2.1). An adequate fluid intake is also important, along with gentle exercise.

Q3.12 Nausea and vomiting are common in early pregnancy. Can diet help?

Morning sickness, nausea and vomiting occur in around half to three-quarters of pregnant women during the first trimester. Consumption of small, frequent meals can help if these symptoms are experienced. Plenty of carbohydrate foods should be encouraged and plenty of fluids. A warm drink and a dry biscuit or dry toast may also be helpful.

Q3.13 What about cravings?

During pregnancy, it is not unusual to have cravings for certain foods and aversions to other foods. The cause of aversions and cravings during pregnancy is uncertain. It may be a result of altered taste perceptions. As long as a healthy, varied diet is being consumed, there should not be cause for concern. Once the baby has been born, tastes usually return to normal.

Sometimes cravings are experienced for non-food substances, such as chalk or soap; this is known as pica. The incidence of pica has decreased in recent years in the UK.

Q3.14 Are there problems associated with eating a vegetarian or vegan diet during pregnancy?

Pregnancy places extra nutritional demands on the body and, for those following a restricted diet, extra care may be needed to ensure that nutritional intake is adequate. As the diet becomes more restrictive, e.g. a vegan diet (see Q4.18–4.21), obtaining sufficient intakes of some micronutrients may become difficult. Mean intakes of calcium, iodine, vitamin B_{12} and riboflavin have been reported to be low in non-pregnant vegan women, so there may be a need to focus on these nutrients in particular (see British Nutrition Foundation, 1995). Vegan diets may also be bulky. An increase in foods that are energy and nutrient dense (i.e. a high nutrient:energy ratio) should overcome any problems.

However, provided that the diets of vegetarian and vegan women are well planned (and the woman enters pregnancy adequately nourished), dietary intake should be adequate to meet nutritional requirements throughout pregnancy.

Q3.15 Is there any special dietary advice for pregnant teenagers?

England has one of the highest teenage conception rates in the developed world and the highest in western Europe (Department of Health, 1999). For a teenage body that is not fully developed, pregnancy can be very demanding. Special help and advice may be needed to ensure that nutritional intake meets requirements, particularly for nutrients such as iron and calcium. A nutrient-dense diet should be promoted, which takes account of any particular food preferences. It may also be necessary to provide information about achieving a balanced diet within a restricted income, if finances are a problem (see Q3.70 and Q3.105).

Q3.16 Should women of Asian origin be given special advice regarding
vitamin D?

It is quite common for Asian women to have a low-birthweight baby.
This is partly determined by short stature and low pre-pregnancy
weight. However, ensuring adequate weight gain during pregnancy
may be important for some women (see Table 3.2).

Asian women who choose to cover their skin when outdoors or
who spend little time outdoors may benefit from specific advice on
vitamin D. This vitamin is important for the uptake and utilisation of
calcium, needed in the calcification of the fetal skeleton in the latter
stages of pregnancy. The major source of this vitamin is via synthesis
in skin exposed to sunlight. The darker skin of Asian women reduces
the access to the UV light needed to catalyse this reaction and this
may exacerbate the problem, although vitamin D deficiency (which
manifests in osteomalacia in adults and rickets in children) is not
seen to be a problem in African-Caribbean women, for example.

Some vitamin D is naturally available from food, e.g. oil-rich fish,
eggs and meat, and it is added by law to margarine. It is also added
voluntarily to low-fat spreads and breakfast cereals. During pregnancy, however, it is recommended that all women should receive
supplementary vitamin D to achieve an intake of 10 μg/day. This
may be particularly important for women who receive little sunlight
exposure and also for vegetarians, who have a narrower range of
vitamin D-containing foods from which to choose.

Q3.17 What advice should be offered with regard to liver intake?

Liver is a rich source of a number of nutrients, including iron and
folic acid. However, it is now recognised that liver can also contain
very high concentrations of vitamin A, which can be harmful to a
developing baby during the early stages of pregnancy. For this
reason, women who are pregnant or who may become pregnant
should avoid liver and foods made from liver, such as pâté (see Q3.1).

Q3.18 What is toxoplasmosis?

Toxoplasmosis is caused by a parasite found in raw meat, cat faeces
and occasionally in unpasteurised goats' milk. In rare cases, the
infection can be passed on to an unborn baby and cause eye and

brain damage. A high regard for food hygiene is therefore very important for pregnant women (see Q5.16). In particular, they should avoid eating raw or uncooked meat, unpasteurised goats' milk or goats' cheese, or unwashed fruit and vegetables. After handling raw meat, chopping boards, utensils and hands should be washed thoroughly. When gardening or emptying cat litter trays, rubber gloves should always be worn.

> Q3.19 Is there anything that can be done to guard against infection with bacteria such as *Listeria monocytogenes*, *Salmonella* spp. and *Escherichia coli*?

Again, good food hygiene practices are very important (see Q5.16). In addition, special dietary advice is relevant during pregnancy.

Listeriosis is a rare condition in the UK; however, it can harm an unborn child. Consequently, pregnant women should avoid those foods in which high levels of the listeria bacteria have, on occasions, been found, including all types of pâté, and soft and blue-veined varieties of cheese (there is no risk with other types of cheese, e.g. hard cheeses such as Cheddar, cheese spread or cottage cheese, because the bacteria cannot survive). Any pre-prepared foods should be heated until piping hot, and should not be eaten cold. Fruit and vegetables should be washed well, especially if they are to be eaten raw. All foods should be stored according to instructions.

Poultry and eggs are foods particularly associated with *Salmonella* bacteria, and pregnant women should therefore be careful when handling these foods and adopt good hygienic practices. In addition, raw egg or uncooked eggs should not be eaten, and eggs should be cooked until both the white and yolk are solid. All meat, especially poultry, should be cooked thoroughly and raw meat should not be allowed to come into contact with or drip on to other food.

E. coli poisoning can also be harmful and is again best avoided through good hygienic practices, particularly when handling raw meat.

> Q3.20 Some women are concerned about their intake of pesticides or additives. What advice can be offered?

Additives permitted for use in foods in the UK undergo the most stringent safety tests over a long period of time before being approved. Additives used in foods are safe for consumption, only a very small minority of people being sensitive or allergic to additives (see Q1.13). There should be no need to avoid food additives during pregnancy.

In recent years, there has been increasing interest in organic foods, as a result of concerns about pesticide levels in food (see Q5.15). It is reassuring to note that the Ministry of Agriculture, Food and Fisheries (MAFF) conduct regular analyses of food samples to ensure that foods are pesticide free. In 1997, for example, 70% of food samples analysed by MAFF for their pesticide residue content were found to be residue free, and 29% contained levels below the maximum residue level (MRL). The MRL is the maximum level expected to be found in a sample and is the legal standard against which residues are measured. The MRL is not the same as the acceptable daily intake (ADI). Even if someone were to consume large amounts of foods containing the MRL, they would not be expected to reach the ADI, because a large margin of safety is incorporated. The ADI takes into account vulnerable groups such as children and elderly people.

Nutrition and Breast-feeding

Q3.21 What is the prevalence of breast-feeding these days?

Detailed information on the prevalence of breast-feeding can be found in the regular national surveys conducted by the Office of Population Censuses and Surveys (OPCS). The incidence reached an all-time low in the 1960s. The most recent survey indicated that 63% of mothers in the UK started to breast-feed but, by 6 weeks, 39% of those who had started had stopped (White et al., 1992). However, because use of supplementary bottles of infant formula is now commonplace, by 4 weeks of age, most babies were receiving at least some infant formula, and by 4 months three-quarters were fully bottle-fed. There is a strong influence of social class on the incidence of breast-feeding: 89% of mothers of first babies in social class I, compared with 50% of first-time mothers in social class V. Women who have stayed in full-time education after age 18 and older women are also more likely to breast-feed (White et al., 1992).

Q3.22 Which aspects of diet are particularly important for women who are breast-feeding?

It has been calculated that breast-feeding carries a daily energy cost of 650 kcal. However, some of this is obtained by using up fat stored during pregnancy for this purpose. Consequently, women who exclusively breast-feed for 3–4 months need an extra 500 kcal/day, on average, which corresponds to an average milk output of 750 ml/day.

Assuming that this extra energy is obtained via consumption of a balanced and varied diet, the additional needs for essential vitamins and minerals will also be met. Additional requirements for calcium are particularly high: an extra 550 mg/day are needed (equivalent to just over an extra three-quarters of a pint of milk), bringing the total RNI to 1250 mg/day (1350 mg/day for women under 18 years). Table 3.3 shows the increase in nutritional requirements that occurs during lactation.

Vitamin D is also important; it is needed for absorption of calcium (see Q2.22).

Table 3.3 Daily nutrient requirements during lactation

	Lactation (0–4 months)[b]	Lactation (beyond 4 months)[b]
Energy (kcal)	+450–570[a]	+480[a]
Protein (g)	+11	+8
Thiamin (mg)	+0.2	+0.2
Riboflavin (mg)	+0.5	+0.5
Niacin (mg)	+2	+2
Vitamin B12 (µg)	+0.5	+0.5
Folate (µg)	+60	+60
Vitamin C (mg)	+30	+30
Vitamin A (µg)	+350	+350
Vitamin D (µg)	10	10
Calcium (mg)	+550	+550
Phosphorus (mg)	+440	+440
Magnesium (mg)	+50	+50
Zinc (mg)	+6.0	+2.5
Copper (mg)	+0.3	+0.3
Selenium (µg)	+15	+15
Iron (mg)	No increment	No increment

[a]Assuming that weaning is begun at 3–4 months, if breast milk remains the sole source of nourishment, an extra 90 kcal/day will be needed.
[b]See Tables 1.1–1.3 for pre-pregnancy needs.

Although maternal diet has virtually no effect on the protein, total fat and energy composition of breast milk, the fatty acid composition of a woman's diet will influence the fatty acid profile of her milk, and this may prove to be of importance, especially with regard to the amount of essential fatty acids present (see Q2.4). These are needed for brain development, for example.

If a woman's diet is poor during pregnancy and breast-feeding, her own stores will be reduced so as not to compromise the baby's growth. It is important, therefore, that women are encouraged to eat healthily between pregnancies as well as during pregnancy, especially if babies are born close together.

Q3.23 What is colostrum and how does the composition of milk change, both during a feed and as the baby grows?

Colostrum is the first milk produced after the baby is born. It is of a different composition to the milk that follows (Table 3.4, page 64) and is particularly rich in protective factors and growth factors. As well as changing in composition over time, breast milk also changes in composition during a feed. The milk available at the start of a feed is richer in nutrients and energy.

Q3.24 What are the health advantages to mother and baby of breast-feeding?

Breast milk is the ideal combination of nutrients designed to meet the infant's needs, and the composition automatically changes as the baby grows. It is also the vehicle for an array of protective factors such as immunoglobulins and growth factors (e.g. enzymes and hormones), which may influence the child's development. It enables the infant to regulate his or her own food intake and it is cheap, hygienic and convenient. Exclusive breast-feeding for 6 weeks or more may also help protect against gastrointestinal and respiratory infections, and development of allergies (see British Nutrition Foundation, 1997, 2000).

From the mother's point of view, breast-feeding aids involution of the uterus and may help in the loss of surplus body fat. However, this is not the time for reducing energy intake in order to lose weight.

Q3.25 How do modern infant formulas compare with breast milk?

Nutritionally, infant formulas are now very close to the composition of breast milk. However, they cannot as yet provide the anti-infection

Table 3.4 Nutrient composition of colostrum and mature human milk (per 100g)

	Human milk: colostrum	Human milk: mature
Energy, kcal	56	69
Carbohydrate (g)	6.6	7.2
Fat (g)	2.6	4.1
Protein (g)	2.0	1.3[a]
Thiamin (mg)	Tr	0.02
Riboflavin (mg)	0.03	0.03
Niacin (mg)	0.05	0.22
Vitamin B12 (μg)	0.1	0.01
Folate (μg)	2	5
Vitamin C (mg)	7	4
Vitamin A (retinol) (μg)	155	58
Vitamin D (μg)	–	0.04
Calcium (mg)	28	34
Phosphorus (mg)	14	15
Magnesium (mg)	3	3
Zinc (mg)	0.6	0.3
Copper (mg)	0.05	0.04
Selenium (μg)	–	1
Iron (mg)	0.07	0.07

[a]N × 6.38. Excluding the non-protein nitrogen, true protein = 0.85 g/100 g.

and growth factors present in breast milk or convey the immunological properties. The nutritional composition of infant formulas is governed by an EC Directive. Two types of standard infant formulas are available – whey-dominant and casein-dominant. Whey-dominant milks are manufactured from dialysed whey protein obtained from cows' milk and casein-dominant milks are based on whole cows' milk protein. Usually, babies start on a whey-dominant formula, but there is no evidence that this is more beneficial than a casein-dominant milk, although the higher calcium:phosphorus ratio in whey-dominant milks may be more appropriate for very young babies. Formula milks are fortified with vitamins A and D.

Infants on breast milk have a similar growth rate to today's bottle-fed infants. As research provides more information on the significance of components of breast milk, e.g. long chain fatty acids and the amino acid taurine (both important for brain and retinal development), consideration is being given to the addition of these to formula milks.

Q3.26 What is the current advice on the use of soya-based formulas?

Soya formulas are sometimes considered as an alternative for babies identified as allergic to cows' milk proteins; however, many babies who react to cows' milk protein also react to soya formula. Some studies have suggested that as many as 40% of infants may be affected, although a more conservative estimate is 5–10% (MacDonald, 1995). Current advice is that, although soya-based formulas are designed for use from birth, they should not be used as the first choice unless there is a specific reason for excluding formulas based on cows' milk, e.g. the child is being fed a vegan diet (see Q3.45). They are not a reliable alternative for a child with cows' milk allergy who may also develop an allergic response to soya. For such children, the best option is one of the formulas based on hydrolysed protein, which are available on prescription.

Q3.27 Do pre-term infants have special needs and how may these be met?

Babies born prematurely require extra nutrients for rapid growth (the same applies to other low-birthweight infants). Pre-term infants are at a special disadvantage because they have missed the period of maximum transfer of energy and nutrients that occurs during the last months of pregnancy. In addition, the immature state of their gastrointestinal system and kidneys results, respectively, in poorer absorption and reduced retention of nutrients.

Before discharge from hospital, pre-term babies will have received either a pre-term formula, designed to meet their needs, or a combination of breast milk and pre-term formula. For small infants, a pre-term formula may be used on discharge, but usually babies are able to progress to a standard formula or continue on breast milk. Pre-term formulas have a higher nutrient density. Even after discharge, pre-term infants will require iron and vitamin supplements.

Q3.28 Should women who are breast-feeding avoid any particular foods?

Some women report that, after they have consumed certain foods, e.g. spicy foods or onions, their babies experience abdominal discomfort. If this occurs, such foods should perhaps be avoided, provided omission of the trigger foods does not result in an unbalanced diet.

Alcohol should largely be avoided during lactation, because of the risk to the baby. Non-nutritive substances such as caffeine, nicotine and other amines and alkaloids can pass into breast milk, and heavy consumption of coffee, tea and cola drinks has been reported to cause restlessness in some infants (Lawrence, 1989). With regard to the prevention of allergy or other food intolerance in the baby, the benefits of mothers avoiding specific foods during pregnancy and lactation are not proven. Furthermore, exposure via the mother may be an important factor in establishing a normal immune response to proteins in the diet. Avoidance of foods associated with allergic reactions, e.g. milk, eggs or nuts, should be seriously considered only when there is a strong family history of atopy (see Q3.10).

Q3.29 Is fluid intake important?

An adequate fluid intake is crucial postpartum for establishing breast-feeding and remains important throughout, given that, by 2–3 months of age, a baby may be taking as much as 820 ml of milk a day. The best guide to requirement is thirst, and forced drinking of extra fluid will not increase milk quality or quantity.

Q3.30 What is a normal weight gain for a breast-fed baby and does it differ if a baby is bottle-fed?

Modern infant formulas result in a similar weight gain and growth trajectory to that seen with breast milk. However, breast-fed babies tend to be longer and thinner than bottle-fed babies. New growth charts, available from the Child Growth Foundation (London) (see Useful addresses), have recently been developed. The birthweight of a healthy baby generally doubles in the first 4–5 months, and triples by 1 year.

Q3.31 Do breast-fed babies need vitamin supplements?

Vitamin supplements (A, C and D) are recommended from 6 months of age for babies who are not bottle-fed. However, if there is any doubt about the vitamin status of a baby under 6 months, e.g. an infant breast-fed by a poorly nourished mother, vitamin drops can be given from 1 month. Formula milks are already supplemented with these nutrients.

Q3.32 Do breast-fed babies need fluid other than milk in the first few months?

Supplementary feeds of infant formula can hinder the establishment and maintenance of breast-feeding. Special baby drinks are also unnecessary for both breast- and bottle-fed infants. Even in hot weather, extra water or glucose solutions are not necessary before 6 months of age.

Q3.33 What about breast-feeding and AIDS?

The current advice is that HIV-infected women and women with AIDS should not breast-feed their babies (UNAIDS, 1998).

Q3.34 Are there other conditions that make breast-feeding an inappropriate choice?

Women who receive drugs for long-term illnesses or who are drug abusers need to be advised against breast-feeding because many drugs can pass into breast milk.

Babies with severe physical difficulties, e.g. cleft palate, may find breast-feeding difficult, although not impossible. Also very-low-birthweight babies or those who are particularly ill may experience difficulties in breast-feeding. Mothers should be encouraged to discuss feeding methods with their health visitor, doctor or breast-feeding counsellor.

Weaning

Q3.35 Do young babies need drinks other than milk?

Up until the age of 6 months, no drink other than breast or formula milk is needed by a healthy baby (see Q3.32). After this time, boiled unflavoured tap water can be offered. Special baby drinks are not necessary and it is not appropriate to offer babies fizzy drinks, even effervescent water. If still bottled water is used, again it should be boiled and it should be noted that some brands have a relatively high sodium content.

Q3.36 Does it matter which type of water is used to make up feeds or offered as a drink?

Boiled tap water from the cold tap is fine. There is no need to consider bottled water, and effervescent water should never be used for babies. If in an emergency bottled water is used, choose one with a low sodium content and boil it first.

Q3.37 At what age should a baby start to receive solids?

The introduction of solids becomes necessary to meet the changing nutritional needs of a growing baby, to encourage the development of the ability to bite and chew, and to encourage the transition to family foods. The Department of Health advises that most babies do not need solids (anything other than breast or formula milk) before 4 months of age, but that the majority should be offered a mixed diet not later than 6 months of age (Department of Health, 1994c).

Before the age of 4 months, babies find it difficult to pass food from the front to the back of their mouths and some babies do not readily develop the ability to bite and chew before this age. Young babies are also less willing to experiment with new flavours, textures and consistency. Furthermore, the premature introduction of solids may provoke allergy because the immature gut may not be fully able to exclude absorption of foreign proteins (see Q3.49).

Late weaning (after 6 months) is also inadvisable because, by this age, babies accustomed only to liquids may find it more difficult to accept solids, and important developmental stages will have been missed. Also, nutritional status may have been compromised, e.g. iron stores established before birth become depleted by 6 months in breast-fed infants.

Despite this advice, the early introduction of solids is still common in Britain. For example in the 1990 OPCS survey published in 1992 (White et al., 1992), 19% of mothers had introduced solids before 10 weeks of age, and by three months of age, 68% of babies were receiving solids (White et al., 1992). Early introduction was less common in higher social class mothers and in breast-fed infants.

Q3.38 Which foods should be offered first?

In the past, it has been recommended that new foods should be introduced to a baby very gradually, but current advice is that the weaning diet should diversify as soon as possible (Department of Health, 1994c).

Most foods can be tried from 4 months: there are no hard and fast rules. However, babies should not be given chilli and spices (although mildly spiced foods will often be tolerated). Sugar and salt should not be added to foods meant for babies – they are unnecessary (see Q2.2). Whole or chopped nuts should not be given because they can cause choking. As a result of concerns about salmonella poisoning, soft-boiled eggs should not be given (see Q3.19). Eggs should be cooked until both the yolk and white are solid.

Although, the COMA Report on Weaning (Department of Health, 1994c) recommended that pâté and Brie-type cheeses should be avoided until 1 year of age, because of concerns about listeriosis (see Q3.19) this advice has now been retracted.

One of the main aims of weaning is to familiarise a baby with taking food from a spoon, and the first foods offered should have a smooth consistency and bland taste.

Once a baby is 4 months old, the following foods are good ones to try:

- Vegetable or fruit purée, e.g. potato, carrot, yam, plantain, broccoli, banana, apple.
- Non-wheat infant cereals or thin porridge (made from rice, tapioca, cornmeal, sago or millet).
- Puréed lentils (dahl); mild spices may be added.

Once the baby has become used to taking food from a spoon, the variety can be expanded to include well-puréed meat, plain yoghurt (unsweetened, but fruit purée could be added) or custard. Salty foods, such as canned or packet soups or sauces, should be avoided (see Q2.28 and Q3.48).

Commercial baby foods are not essential, but can be convenient, particularly early on (e.g. with powdered products, tiny quantities can be mixed at a time).

Throughout weaning, milk (breast or formula) remains a dominant part of a baby's diet. Babies aged 4–6 months should still have at least 600 ml of breast milk or infant formula each day.

For babies who are breast-fed, iron-fortified commercial baby foods can be particularly useful, because surveys indicate that many infants and preschool children develop a poor iron status (Department of Health, 1994c).

From 6 to 9 months, as the quantity of solid food increases, the baby becomes less dependent on milk feeds to provide energy and nutrients. However, most babies still need 500–600 ml/day. Babies of this age will tolerate stronger tastes, and different textures (e.g. lumpier purées) should be encouraged, as well as expansion of the variety of foods offered. Gluten-containing foods can now be introduced (see Q3.39). Soft finger foods, such as cheese, chopped hard-boiled egg, raw soft fruit (e.g. banana, melon, tomato) and cooked vegetables (e.g. carrot, green beans), can be given and will help develop hand-to-mouth coordination. Small quantities of cows' milk can be introduced after 6 months to mix cereals and make puddings, and a cup or beaker can be introduced. Parents should be advised to provide the following, each day: two to three (small) servings of starchy foods, e.g. bread, potatoes, cereal, rice or pasta; two servings of fruit/vegetables; one serving of meat, fish, beans, lentils or well-cooked egg. Savoury, rather than sweet foods should be encouraged, and salt or sugar should not be added.

Babies aged 9–12 months should be eating three meals a day with snacks and/or drinks of breast milk/formula between meals. Most infants will still need 500–600 ml breast milk or infant formula daily. Foods should generally be of a normal adult texture, but will probably need to be chopped. Parents should aim to provide three to four servings of starchy foods and wholemeal varieties can be included; three to four servings of fruit/vegetables; and diluted unsweetened orange juice may be given with meals (this helps iron absorption from non-haem sources). At least one serving of animal protein (e.g. meat, fish, egg) should be provided daily, plus two servings of vegetable protein (e.g. bread, pulses, cereals). Finger foods remain important and should be included with each meal to encourage self-feeding. Salty foods should be avoided, and biscuits, cakes and other foods with added sugar kept to a minimum (see Q2.2, Q2.28 and Q3.48).

Q3.39 When can gluten-containing foods be introduced?

Gluten is a component of the protein found in wheat and it is present in many foods, particularly bread, pasta and wheat-based breakfast cereals. Gluten sensitivity is the cause of coeliac disease (see Q4.36–4.40). Although the vast majority of babies will be able to tolerate gluten from the onset of weaning, it is recommended that wheat-based foods are not introduced until 6 months of age, as a precaution, particularly where there is a family history of allergic disease. Infant foods designed to be used as early weaning foods are usually gluten free. Alternative cereals include rice and rice-based baby cereal.

Q3.40 Can a microwave be used to sterilise or heat up a feed?

This form of heating is not recommended for bottles of formula. It can result in hot spots, i.e. the heating is not uniform throughout the liquid.

Q3.41 When can cows' milk be introduced?

The Department of Health (1994c) recommends that cows' milk should not be introduced as a main drink until a child is a year old. However, small quantities can be included as part of the weaning diet from 6 months of age, e.g. to mix infant cereals or as custard, milk pudding or cheese sauce. Yoghurt, fromage frais and grated cheese are also acceptable nutrient-rich foods from this age.

Q3.42 What about other drinks?

Fizzy drinks are not suitable for babies (see Q3.35). The same applies to drinks containing artificial sweeteners. In addition, milk feeds, plain water or dilute pure orange juice can be given. The last is a good drink to accompany meals that provide non-haem sources of iron, e.g. pulses, green vegetables and bread, because the vitamin C provided by the orange juice enhances iron absorption (see Q2.20). Such drinks can be offered in a beaker or cup from 6 months of age. The transition to a beaker from this age is important both for developmental reasons and, in the case of sweetened drinks and fruit juices, in relation to good dental practice.

Q3.43 At what age should a cup be introduced?

Use of a cup should be encouraged from 6 months of age (Department of Health, 1994c). By this time, most babies are able to sip rather than just suck, and so the cup or beaker should begin to take over from a bottle, particularly when drinks other than milk, e.g. water, are offered. Currently, some young children continue to have drinks from a bottle into the third or fourth years of life, and this can be associated with several problems (see Q3.100):

- Consumption of large volumes of fluid (possibly of relatively low nutrient density) which can reduce appetite at meal times, resulting in both a poorer nutrient intake and delayed progression to a mixed diet.
- Poor dental health where sweetened drinks are provided in a bottle. Unlike drinks in beakers or cups, which tend to be consumed relatively quickly, children may intermittently suck on a bottle for several hours. Not only does this mean that teeth are exposed to a sugary liquid for a longer period, but also the process of sucking, compared with sipping, causes the liquid to interact differently with the teeth, increasing the risk of damage to developing teeth (see Q2.2).
- Delayed acquisition of food-handling skills and speech.

Q3.44 Why is there concern about the iron (and zinc) intake of babies and
        young children?

Babies born at full term have a store of iron that is sufficient for the first 6 months of life. Breast milk provides quite low levels of iron, although what is contained is well absorbed. One of the reasons weaning by 6 months is important is that the baby needs additional sources of iron once its own stores became depleted.

The richest source of well-absorbed iron available is red meat, but many mothers choose not to introduce this as a weaning food, partly because of the difficulties associated with puréeing meat. Although foods that provide iron include pulses, green vegetables, bread and fortified breakfast cereals, these may not be major items in the child's diet. As an alternative, manufactured weaning foods are often iron fortified and formula milk routinely contains iron. Poor iron status results in anaemia, but has also been linked with reduced cognitive function.

Zinc is found in some of the same foods as iron – meat is a particularly important source (see Q2.29). So, if babies are receiving a low iron intake, their diet may also be low in zinc. One of the problems associated with poor zinc status is an increased susceptibility to infection.

In the UK, iron-deficiency anaemia in toddlers is the most commonly reported nutritional disorder of early childhood. A recent survey of preschool children indicated that 12% of children aged 1.5–2.5 years and 6% of children aged 2.5–3.5 years are anaemic (Gregory et al., 1995). In 3.5–4.5 year olds, the prevalence was 4% of boys and 8% of girls.

Directly as a result of the concern about the prevalence of low iron intakes, guidance has been issued by the Government's advisory committee, COMA, that babies up to the age of 12 months should receive either breast milk or an infant formula that is fortified with iron, to guarantee their iron intake (Department of Health, 1994c). It is also important that iron-rich weaning foods are included in the diet from 4 months of age onwards. Cows' milk can be introduced as a main drink from the age of 12 months, but can be used as a component of the weaning diet from, say, 6 months onwards, e.g. to mix infant cereal or in custard or cheese sauce (see Q3.41).

Q3.45 What advice should be offered to mothers who wish to feed a vegetarian diet?

Young children have high requirements for energy (calories) and nutrients in relation to their capacity for food and so are particularly at risk of nutritional deficiencies if they are fed a restricted diet.

Mothers who want their children to follow a vegetarian or vegan diet should be encouraged to breast-feed, and in this respect it is particularly important that the mother herself is adequately nourished, especially if she plans to breast-feed for a year or more (as often happens with vegan mothers). As with other breast-fed infants, vitamin supplements should be given from 6 months of age (or earlier if the mother's diet is thought to be inadequate). For mothers who choose to bottle-feed, standard infant formulas are suitable for vegetarians and, for vegan babies, soya-based infant formulas are available (see Q3.26 and Q3.31). Ordinary soya milk is not suitable. As a result of concerns about the sugar content, from 6 months of age, soya formula should be confined to meal times (500–600 ml/day) and ideally provided in a cup.

The weaning diet should be as varied as possible and follow the guidelines given above. For children following a vegan or other diet in which the choice of foods is restricted, particular attention needs to be paid to balance and diversity (see Q4.21). By the end of the first year, babies should be eating four servings daily from the cereals group and the fruit/vegetables group. At least two servings from the milk/milk products group (in addition to milk feeds) should be consumed by children on a vegetarian diet, and vegan children should have similar quantities of soya cheese or yoghurt. Some of these products are fortified with vitamins and minerals, e.g. calcium, and such varieties are preferable. At least two daily servings of foods considered to be alternatives to meat, fish and poultry should be eaten, i.e. beans, lentils, nut pastes, seed pastes, tofu or textured vegetable protein (TVP).

Ensuring an adequate intake of iron and zinc is particularly important (see Q2.6 and Q2.29).

Q3.46 Does advice to eat more fibre and less fat apply to babies?

Recommendations to eat a diet low in fat and high in fibre do not apply to babies and young children because, at this stage of development, children have a high requirement for nutrients and energy in relation to the quantity of food that they can consume, and such diets tend to be bulky and filling, with individual foods having a low nutrient density. Fat provides more than twice as many calories as protein or carbohydrate and this is reflected in the contribution fat makes to the energy content of breast milk. Nevertheless, during the first year or so of life a baby's diet moves from one relatively rich in fat to one with a relative abundance of carbohydrate. Low-fat foods, high-fibre cereals and wholemeal bread can be included in a young child's diet, but parents should be dissuaded from implementing a low-fat/high-fibre diet before the age of 2 years; after this age, provided the child is eating a good range of foods and has a good appetite, a gradual transition can, however, be made (Department of Health, 1994c). Children should continue on whole milk as a main drink until at least 2 years of age (5 years if the child is a poor eater). Semi-skimmed milk can be introduced at 2 years of age, but fully skimmed milk is not appropriate for children under the age of 5 because of its low energy content and the absence of vitamin A (which is present only in the cream).

Q3.47 What is the advice on sugar intake?

Appreciation of sweetness is an acquired taste that is not present at birth. Therefore, although weaning foods may taste bland to parents, there is no need to add sugar to foods or drinks. As children progress on to a mixed diet, sweet foods and drinks are best reserved for mealtimes because it is the frequency rather than the amount of sugar consumed that influences dental health (see Q2.2). Between meals, water or milk is the best drink from a dental health point of view. Sweetened drinks at bedtime are particularly associated with poor dental health (Gregory and Hinds, 1995; Gregory et al., 1995). A dental survey of children aged 1.5–4.5 years revealed that almost one in five children (17%) had some form of tooth decay (Gregory and Hinds, 1995).

The prevalence of tooth decay rose from 4% in 1.5–2.5 year olds to 30% in 3.5–4.5 year olds. A north/south gradient existed, with the prevalence being higher in the north. Dental caries was also more likely in low-income households. More information on oral health can be found in a British Nutrition Foundation Task Force Report on this subject (British Nutrition Foundation, 1999b).

Q3.48 What is the advice on giving salt to babies and young children?

The kidneys of babies are immature and unable to excrete salt efficiently. For this reason, salt should never be added to foods given to them. Even for toddlers, addition of salt to foods is unnecessary and salty foods should be strictly moderated because their regular consumption can lead to the acquisition of a taste for salt, which in the long term may increase the chances of raised blood pressure developing (see Q2.28).

Q3.49 What advice should be given to families with a history of allergic disease?

In the early months of life, the relatively immature gut is far more likely than later in life to allow an intact food protein to cross the gut mucosa and travel into the bloodstream. In predisposed infants, development of a food allergy can be the outcome. Indeed, most cases of food allergy occur in young children and the majority outgrow their allergies within 12–24 months, i.e. before school age (see Q4.25). The most common allergies are to those foods encountered in the early months, i.e. milk, egg and, these days, soya. The chances of sensitisation are greatest in the first few months, hence the recommendation to delay weaning until 4 months. Where there is a history of allergic disease in a family, mothers are usually advised to breast-feed exclusively for 4–6 months. This is thought to offer some protection against allergy. In such children, weaning before 4 months should be actively discouraged and ideally delayed until closer to 6 months. First weaning foods should be those least likely to result in allergies, i.e. non-wheat cereals (e.g. rice-based cereal foods), fruit and vegetables. Parents should also be advised to limit exposure to non-food allergens, e.g. pet hair and house dust mites. Where an allergy is suspected, expert advice should always be sought before foods are eliminated from the diet. Random eliminations can result in growth faltering and nutrient deficiencies.

The benefits of a woman avoiding specific foods during pregnancy or breast-feeding in order to reduce the chances of allergy developing in her baby have not been demonstrated convincingly. Furthermore, omitting such foods may inadvertently result in dietary inadequacies, and may deny the baby (or fetus) the ability to develop natural tolerance, via its mother, to these food proteins. (See Q3.9, Q3.10 and Q3.28.)

Q3.50 How common is allergy in young children?

Food allergy is a specific type of food intolerance and most often affects young children, the prevalence being highest among the very young at around 5–7%. However, the majority of sufferers (around 80–90%) outgrow their sensitivity by the age of 3 years (see British Nutrition Foundation, 2000). In other age groups, the prevalence is less, being 1–2% in children and less than 1% in adults. Most children outgrow their allergy within 12–24 months and so most are allergy free when they start school. An exception to this is peanut allergy which tends to persist into adulthood (see Q4.23–4.34). Food allergy and other adverse reactions to food are the subject of a British Nutrition Foundation Task Force, which is due to report in 2001.

Q3.51 Should vitamin supplements be recommended?

A survey of children aged 1.5–4.5 years in different regions of the UK during 1992–3 demonstrated a need for vitamin D supplementation at least in the winter months for susceptible groups, such as those living in northern Britain and Asian children (Gregory et al., 1995). The 'cover up' policy encouraged to reduce skin exposure to sunlight and protect against skin cancer may compromise the vitamin D status of young children. The same study found that 12% of British children aged 1.5–4.5 have low blood levels of retinol (vitamin A). The recommendation on supplementation for infants and children is to take supplement drops containing vitamins A, C and D from 6 months until 2 years of age. Where there is local evidence of an inadequate intake of these vitamins, supplements should be continued until the age of 5 years.

Nutrition and Preschool Children

Q3.52 Are there any particular nutritional considerations for preschool children?

The most prevalent nutritional deficiency in this age group is iron-deficiency anaemia which affects cognitive performance and behaviour (see Q2.6 and Q3.44).

A survey of preschool children published in 1995 (Gregory et al., 1995) indicated that other considerations for this age group are:

- dental health
- supply of sufficient calories
- poor dietary variety
- faddy eating
- vitamin D status in some subgroups.

Q3.53 Does advice to eat more fibre and less fat apply to preschool children?

This advice does not apply to children under the age of 2 years (see Q1.8). However, from the age of 2, among children who have a good appetite and eat a good range of foods, this advice can gradually be implemented. The process needs to be gradual because a low-fat, high-fibre diet can be very bulky and may preclude sufficient food being consumed to ensure that all nutrient needs are met. Semi-skimmed milk can be introduced at the age of 2, but skimmed milk is not appropriate for the under-5s because of the absence of vitamin A (found in the cream) and its low energy content. Bran-enriched foods should be avoided because their high phytate content can block absorption of minerals such as iron and possibly calcium.

> Q3.54 What advice should be offered to the mothers of children who are faddy
> eaters?

Faddy eating patterns are common among young children as eating habits and preferences for foods start to develop. Although food refusal can be distressing for parents, it is a normal part of a child's development. Children quickly learn that mealtimes can be disrupted by their refusal to eat, but such behaviour is unlikely to have long-term effects on growth and development.

Possible reasons for such behaviour include the following:

- Excessive fluid intake between meals – some children fill themselves up with drinks and have no appetite at meal times (see Q3.43). This can be overcome by not giving drinks within an hour before mealtimes and modulating the amount drunk between meals. If the child is thirsty, water will quench thirst without providing calories.
- Continuous snacking between meals – most young children have small appetites and so nutritious snacks between meals can be a useful and perfectly acceptable way of meeting nutrient needs. But some children can end up eating all their meals as poorly constructed snacks of relatively low nutritional value.
- Suitability of the food and utensils – some children may refuse to eat a meal because the food is not cut into appropriately sized pieces or they cannot manage with the utensils provided.
- The mealtime setting – toddlers can easily be distracted and are unable to concentrate even for short periods. Toys or the television can be big distractions. Some children respond well to new foods if they are encouraged to serve themselves.
- Parents should be encouraged to avoid arguments about food and should never force feed a child. Other ideas include: avoiding punishment but giving plenty of praise when a food is eaten; introducing new or unfamiliar foods without any fuss; establishing regular eating patterns and mealtimes; and making mealtimes fun – letting the child help with preparation of the food or laying the table. If a meal is refused, it should be removed and no more

food offered until the next mealtime. In particular, it is important not to offer sweets, biscuits or other snacks if the meal remained uneaten at mealtime.

Q3.55 What advice should be offered in relation to oral health?

Despite the remarkable reduction in the prevalence of caries in British children over the last 25 years, the National Diet and Health Survey found that 17% of children aged 1.5–4.5 years have dental decay (Gregory and Hinds, 1995). There was a north/south gradient, with a higher prevalence in Scotland than the south of England. Most disease was discovered in children of poor families and where mothers were less well educated. Extrinsic sugars, often in the form of confectionery, table sugar and soft drinks, were found to be the most important dietary factor in the aetiology of dental caries. However, it is the frequency of sugar consumption, rather than the amount, that appears to be the most crucial factor (see Q2.2). It is therefore recommended to confine the consumption of sugar-containing foods and drinks to mealtimes. The regular use of a fluoride toothpaste offers considerable protection against a sugar challenge. (For further information see British Nutrition Foundation Task Force on Oral Health, 1999b.)

Another concern is dental erosion (also known as tooth tissue loss). Paediatric dentists believe this to be on the increase in children (see British Nutrition Foundation, 1999b), but this cannot be verified owing to the lack of longitudinal data. The survey mentioned above showed a prevalence of 13% in 3.5–4.5 year olds. In 5–6 year olds the prevalence has been reported to be 25% (O'Brien, 1994). Erosion of dental enamel results from chemical attack by acids other than those produced by the plaque bacteria. It is suspected that fruit juices and drinks, particularly if fed in bottles or reservoir feeders, are contributing to this problem. Dilution of fruit juice helps to some extent by slightly reducing the acidity level (i.e. raising the pH). Fruit juices are important sources of vitamin C but frequent and excessive consumption should be avoided. (See Q3.42–3.43 for advice on foods and drinks to promote dental health.)

Q3.56 When should tooth brushing be started?

As soon as teeth begin to emerge, they can be cleaned with a tiny amount of baby toothpaste or gel, using a small soft brush or a clean handkerchief wrapped around the parent's finger. It is important that no more than a pea-sized piece of toothpaste is used because the child is likely to swallow much of this and ingestion of too much toothpaste can lead to mottling of the teeth as a result of excessive fluoride intake. The Department of Health recommends that parents should brush their children's teeth up to the age of 6–7 years (Department of Health, 1994c).

The British Dental Association recommends that toddlers should make their first visit to the dentist at about 18 months to 2 years of age. The main aim of this visit is to become familiar with the dental environment. The importance of regular check-ups should be stressed.

Q3.57 What is the advice on fluoride?

Dentists may recommend fluoride supplements if the local water supply is not fluoridated. Government advice is that water supplies should be fluoridated to an optimum of one part per million (Department of Health, 1994c) (see Q2.36).

Q3.58 What about vegetarian diets?

As has already been indicated, iron-deficiency anaemia is quite common in preschool children (see Q3.44) and vegetarian diets can potentially be low in iron because of the avoidance of meat (see Q4.21).

The general advice on achieving a balanced diet described earlier and the specific advice given in the section on weaning applies (Q3.45).

Other nutrients that need to be considered for children on a vegetarian diet include vitamin B_{12} and zinc. Intakes of these are likely to be adequate, however, if milk and milk products are consumed. The diets of vegan children may need special attention.

Nutrition and Primary Schoolchildren

Q3.59 What are the nutritional issues for this age group?

The composition of the diet in childhood is important to sustain growth and health in this period of rapid development. Eating habits that help to reduce the risk of chronic disease later in life are best established in childhood. Young children have a high requirement for energy and other nutrients, yet their appetites are relatively small. They therefore require frequent meals consisting of foods that contain energy and nutrients in a relatively concentrated form. A varied diet, which includes plenty of milk and dairy foods, meat, fish, cereals, vegetables and fruit, will provide all the nutrients that a child requires. However, young children frequently exhibit food fads which can last for months or even years and, as a result, the range of foods eaten may be extremely limited. It is therefore vital that the few foods that are eaten contain a variety of nutrients, and are consumed in sufficient amount. Between-meal snacks can be useful to enable children to obtain sufficient energy intake, yet the erratic eating pattern of many young children is often of concern to parents. Although snacking need not be unhealthy, as long as choices are appropriate, the most popular snack foods among young children tend to be high in fat and sugar. Regular consumption of such foods can reduce the appetite at mealtimes and lead to poor nutrient intake (see Q3.44). In addition, the frequent consumption of sticky, sugary snacks can increase the risk of dental caries. Regular meals, combined with healthy snacks, should therefore be encouraged.

The National Diet and Nutrition Survey of young people aged 4–18 years showed that most children have adequate intakes of most vitamins (Gregory et al., 2000), an exception being that 13% of 11–18 year olds had low vitamin D status. Vitamin D is usually provided via exposure to sunlight (see below) and is essential for the development of healthy bones. However, the report indicates that a sizeable proportion of children, particularly older girls, may have inadequate intakes of a number of minerals, including zinc, calcium, magnesium and iron. Foods such as liver and red meat, which provide the best source of easily absorbable iron (haem iron), are sometimes unpopular with children. Many children consume few green vegetables and little fresh fruit, resulting in low vitamin C intakes and poor iron absorption from non-haem sources. Iron-deficiency anaemia is associated with frequent infections, poor weight gain and delay in development (see Q2.6). Calcium is important for the development of strong bones in this age group and foods such as milk and dairy products should be encouraged. Children in low-income families are at greater risk of inadequate nutrient intake and poor growth. The intakes of several vitamins, particularly folate and vitamin C, are lowest in children whose families are claiming benefits, reflecting lower intakes of fruit and vegetables.

Although children's fat intakes are currently close to the population goal of 35% of dietary energy, intakes of saturated fatty acids exceed the recommended population level for adults of 11% of energy, and intakes of sugars and salt are also high in many children (Gregory et al., 2000). Avoiding the frequent consumption of sugary foods and drinks between meals could help to prevent the formation of dental caries (see Q2.2), particularly when dental hygiene is poor. (For more information about the findings of the national report or the public health implications see Smithers et al., 2000 and Buttriss, 2000b, respectively.)

With the exception of the youngest children (4–6 years), children in Britain are largely inactive. About 40% of boys and 60% of girls spend, on average, less than 1 hour a day in activities of at least moderate intensity (Gregory et al., 2000) and therefore fail to meet the Health Education Authority's recommendation for young people's participation in physical activity. For boys and girls in the oldest age group (15–18 years), this proportion increases to 56% and 69% respectively. Unless action is taken to improve physical activity in children, the prevalence of obesity will continue to rise. There may also be implications for vitamin D status if children do not play outside. The best way to prevent weight gain is to encourage daily physical activity and discourage excessive consumption of high-fat and high-sugar foods. However, any treatment of overweight in young children by dietary means needs to be supervised carefully and undertaken gradually, by slowing weight gain, rather than by encouraging weight loss. Drastic dietary manipulation during this period must be avoided and emphasis placed on the adoption of an active lifestyle.

Q3.60 Do school milk schemes still exist?

Subsidised school milk can be made available to children in primary schools via the EC School Milk Subsidy Scheme. This scheme allows children to purchase 250 ml of milk daily (either whole milk or semi-skimmed) at a reduced price. Families in receipt of income support are eligible to receive a free pint of milk a day for every child under 5. Children of low-income families attending a recognised playgroup or nursery are also entitled to a third of a pint of milk, without charge, on each day attended. More information on these schemes is available from the National Dairy Council (5–7 John Princes Street, London W1M 0AP).

Q3.61 What guidance exists on school meals?

Schools often provide children with their first experience of freedom to choose foods solely according to their own preferences. Although food eaten in school constitutes only part of a schoolchild's food intake, it can make an important contribution to the energy and nutrient intake of the overall diet. Although the nutrient composition of school meals can vary widely, they are thought to provide a healthier alternative to food bought from sources such as cafés and take-aways.

Before 1980, school meals had to meet prescribed nutritional standards, providing one-third of the recommended daily energy intake and 40% of the recommended protein intake at that time, as well as some vitamins and minerals. The Education Act of 1980 removed the statutory obligation for schools to provide school meals of a set nutritional standard. Each local education authority became responsible for setting its own standards and the basic requirements were for the provision of a meal for children in receipt of free school meals, and provision of a place for children to eat sandwiches brought to school.

The food provided at lunchtime therefore varies from school to school and from one local education authority to another. At present, most primary schools provide a set meal with some choice of food. This normally includes provision for children who are vegetarian and those who have specific dietary requirements, e.g. for religious reasons. A recent survey of school meals has shown that they are becoming more popular, but a large amount of money is still being spent on snacks, such as carbonated drinks, crisps, sweets/chocolate, on the way to and from school (Gardner Merchant School Meals Survey, 1998). However, the study found that chips were now less popular than jacket potatoes and pizza, and in addition pupils said that they wanted to see more healthy meals and fruit juices on the menu.

Concern about the type of meals provided in schools has led the government to reintroduce compulsory national and quantifiable nutritional standards. These standards will be compulsory in all maintained primary and secondary schools from April 2001 (Department for Education and Employment, 2000a). They promote a healthy balanced diet by encouraging a selection of foods that, over the week, reflects the proportions demonstrated in the *Balance of Good Health* (see Q1.8). Practical guidance to support school food providers in meeting these regulations has been developed (Department for Education and Employment, 2000b).

School meals are particularly important for children of low-income families. Children whose parents receive Income Support or Income-based Jobseeker's Allowance are eligible for free school meals. To encourage uptake of free meals it is important that schemes are put in place in schools to destigmatise recipients, e.g. cashless 'credit' card systems.

Q3.62 What can be done in schools to promote healthier eating habits?

Many factors influence young children's eating habits, including parents and other members of the family, peers and the media. Schools also have an important role to play in equipping children with the skills to prepare food and in the development of their understanding of the need for a healthy diet. Nutrition education in schools provides pupils with opportunities to explore and learn more about diet and health during teaching. The National Curriculum presents a number of opportunities to teach about food and nutrition throughout the school years.

Not all teaching about food and diet occurs, however, as part of specific subject teaching. All occasions where children are eating food in school should provide valuable opportunities for teaching, which include exploration of children's understanding of issues related to food and promoting discussions of diet and health. The need for a 'whole school approach' has been recognised, in which healthy food provision reflects the teaching about food and nutrition in the classroom. Schools should provide a wide choice of food that includes 'healthy' alternatives. School meals should be seen as a tool for nutrition education. Parents need to be informed of the food offered to their children so that they are aware of any nutrients or food groups that may be lacking. Minority groups, such as Asian children, should be suitably catered for.

Some schools provide breakfast and/or snacks and this can be particularly important for those children who have missed breakfast at home or do not have anything on the way to school. The consumption of fruit and vegetables as snacks may be encouraged by making such choices cheaper or having rules about what types of foods can be brought into school and eaten at breaktimes. Promotional events that focus on healthy eating can provide useful opportunities for pupils to taste new foods. Any school projects on food should, however, involve parents.

The national nutritional standards (Department for Education and Employment, 2000a) identify ways in which schools can help to provide a balanced and varied diet using the main food groups (Box 3.1).

Box 3.1 Details of the national standards for school meals

For the purpose of the national standards, food is divided into the following 5 groups:

Group A   fruit and vegetables
Group B   starchy foods
Group C   meat, fish and other non-dairy sources of protein
Group D   milk and dairy foods
Group E   foods containing fat and foods containing sugar

For children who attend nursery schools or nursery units in primary schools:
* foods from each of the first 4 groups (A–D) should be available as part of the lunch.

For pupils of compulsory school age at primary schools:
* foods from each of the first 4 groups (A–D) should be offered each day
* fresh fruit, fruit tinned in juice or fruit salad should be available at least twice a week
* oil-cooked starchy foods from group B (e.g. chips) should be available on no more than 3 days a week
* fish should be served at least once a week
* red meat should be offered at least twice a week
* dairy sources of protein can be included in group C
* recommended portion sizes have been developed.

For pupils at secondary school:
* two types of food from each of the first 4 groups (A–D) should be available each day
* both a fruit and a vegetable should be offered
* at least one of the foods from group B should not be cooked in oil or fat
* fish should be served at least twice a week
* red meat should be available on at least 3 days a week.

Detailed practical advice on how to achieve these objectives is provided (Department for Education and Employment, 2000b), including tips on healthy cooking methods. The guidelines also make a series of suggestions about how school meals should be presented and promoted. Suggestions include:

- modernisation of the image of school meals by reducing queues, improving the image of the eating environment and adoption of high-street style promotional strategies;
- making healthy food appear more attractive by varying colour, texture and flavour, and using garnishes;
- ensuring that healthier foods are prominently displayed;
- offering balanced meals at an attractive price to compete with local traders and introducing customer loyalty discount schemes;
- helping and encouraging pupils to select balanced food choices;
- holding special events such as theme days, which could be linked to the curriculum, or festivals, competitions and prizes;
- taking part in national or local promotions, such as National School Meals Week;
- the inclusion of parents by providing sample meals for parent evenings or inviting parents to come to school for lunch.

Q3.63 Many children take packed lunches. What advice can be given to parents on the composition of these meals?

Packed lunches should be planned to provide variety, balance and moderation in nutrient intakes. A useful guide for a nutritionally balanced packed lunch is to ensure that foods are included from each of the main four food groups – bread/cereals, fruit/vegetables, meat/alternatives and milk/milk products. Examples of suitable foods from each group are shown in Table 3.5

Only when foods from each of the four groups have been included should additional items, such as biscuits or crisps, be considered. Asking children about what they would like and including foods that are fun, as well as healthy, will ensure that the child does not bring his or her lunch home uneaten at the end of the day. Some schools offer parents guidance on how to make packed lunches enjoyable and nutritious.

Table 3.5 Suggested foods from each food group

	Suggestions
Cereal serving	Sandwich, pitta bread, bagel, breadsticks, crackers, chapatti, low sugar scone, currant bun, rice or pasta salad
Fruit/veg serving	Piece of fruit, sticks of raw vegetables e.g. carrots, salad (either in sandwich or separately), unsweetened fruit juice
Milk serving	Small carton of milk, yoghurt, cheese (as sandwich filling or separately)
Meat/alternative serving	Lean meat, canned fish, egg or peanut butter as sandwich filling; hard boiled egg; portion of dahl

Nutrition and Teenagers

Q3.64 What are the nutritional issues for this age group?

The food consumed in adolescence can set the pattern for future food preferences and eating behaviour in adult life, and thus influence long-term health, e.g. establishing appropriate eating habits can help prevent dental caries, obesity, type 2 (non-insulin-dependent) diabetes, cardiovascular disease, bowel problems and osteoporosis (see Q4.1).

The physiological changes occurring during the teenage years, specifically during the time of the adolescent growth spurt, increase the demand for energy and most nutrients. This demand differs between the sexes, with boys requiring more protein and energy than girls as a result of the different rates of growth. However, the growth spurt in girls begins earlier than in boys and girls have their peak requirement for nutrients, on average, about 2 years earlier.

The rapid increase in bone mass during the adolescent growth spurt has a significant impact on the requirement for several nutrients, including protein, phosphorus, vitamin D and calcium. The National Diet and Nutrition Survey showed that around 10% of teenagers have a low blood level of vitamin D and 20% have an inadequate intake of calcium (Gregory et al., 2000); 5% of girls and 12% of boys reported not drinking milk – a major source of calcium in the British diet according to the National Food Survey (MAFF, 2000), providing about 40% of calcium in the diet. An inadequate calcium intake during this period has been associated with a low peak bone mass, a strong predictor of osteoporosis in later life. Although bone mass continues to increase in early adulthood, it is uncertain whether severe deficits in bone mass development during adolescence can be compensated for later. The reference nutrient intake for calcium during adolescence is therefore high: 1000 mg per day for boys and 800 mg for girls (Department of Health, 1991). Absorption of calcium is more efficient, rising to around 40–45% in adolescents compared with about 30% in adults. This can, to some extent, compensate for a low-calcium diet (see Q2.5, Q2.22 and Q3.67).

The teenage years also constitute one of the most vulnerable stages in terms of iron deficiency. Requirements are particularly high for girls, owing to the need to replace losses during menstruation. A substantial proportion of teenagers (14% of girls and 13% of boys aged 15–18 years) have low ferritin levels, suggesting low iron stores (Gregory et al., 2000), and around 3% are estimated to have iron-deficiency anaemia (Prescott-Clarke and Primatesta, 1998). Vegetarian and slimming diets can increase the risk of iron deficiency (see Q2.6 and Q4.20).

Zinc affects protein synthesis and is essential for the growth process (see Q2.29). Low intakes of zinc or diets that are rich in phytate-containing cereals (e.g. unleavened bread), which can inhibit zinc absorption, have been linked to growth retardation and delayed sexual maturation. Low plasma zinc concentrations have been reported during infancy (Department of Health, 1994c) and puberty (Gregory et al., 2000), which are both periods of rapid growth.

Adolescence is a time of increasing independence and a time when school, leisure and social activities are packed into a busy schedule, leaving little time for food and often limited money to spend on it. Eating habits among teenagers are often erratic, with snack foods replacing the conventional eating pattern. Skipping meals, particularly breakfast, becomes more common as children become older (National Dairy Council, 1990). In general, teenagers are getting a disproportionately large amount of their dietary energy from saturated fatty acids and sugar; many are also consuming unhealthy amounts of salt and far too few fruit and vegetables (Gregory et al., 2000). As children grow older, their food choices may be increasingly influenced by external factors such as peer pressure and media-led fashions. A large proportion of advertising targets teenagers. Emotional factors and attitudes to appearance and body image are also important, particularly for girls.

Many older girls and boys are inactive: 56% of boys and 69% of girls are currently failing to meet the Health Education Authority's recommendations for young people of an hour of moderate physical activity per day. Adolescence can be a critical period for the development of obesity, particularly in those who become inactive. There is some evidence that children's weight, cholesterol levels and blood pressure tend to 'track' into adult life (Berenson et al., 1997). Children who are overweight in their early teens are more likely to be overweight as adults and early atherosclerotic plaques have been found in young adults in their early 20s (WHO, 1982). However, there is an increasing tendency, particularly among teenage girls, to control weight by unsuitable methods such as smoking or very-low-calorie diets. In the recent national survey, 16% of the girls aged 15–18 years reported that they were currently dieting to lose weight, compared with 3% of the corresponding group of boys (Gregory et al., 2000). Restriction of food during this period of growth can lead to nutrient deficiencies and problems in later life. Overweight teenagers should therefore be encouraged to increase physical activity rather than go on a diet (see Q4.10).

Q3.65 What can be done to improve dietary variety?

To obtain an adequate nutritional intake, teenagers need to consume a wide variety of foods. Foods from the four main food groups should be included every day. The general principles of a healthy diet apply; teenagers should aim for a diet relatively low in fat, sugar and salt, and high in starchy and fibre-rich foods (Department of Health, 1991). Omission of meals should be discouraged and, although snacks are often necessary to ensure adequate energy intake, a daily pattern of three main meals should be encouraged. Between-meal snacks should be based on foods of high nutrient density, such as bread, toast, sandwiches, breakfast cereal, yoghurt, fresh fruit and vegetables, nuts and milk. Additional items such as confectionery, biscuits, pies, cakes, crisps and soft drinks can also be included, but in moderation.

Q3.66 What can be done to improve iron intake?

Iron is needed for the increases in lean body mass, blood volume and haemoglobin that occur in both sexes and to replace losses during menstruation in girls. Adolescence is recognised to be a vulnerable period in terms of iron deficiency. Teenagers who are slimming or adopting a vegetarian diet may have a very low iron intake. For advice on iron-rich foods, see Q2.6. Iron-fortified breakfast cereals and bread may be particularly useful for vegetarians.

Q3.67 What can be done to improve calcium intake?

The rapid increase in bone mass in adolescence means that there is a higher requirement for calcium than in adults. Boys should aim for 1000 mg of calcium per day and girls for 800 mg (see Table 1.3). In the light of these high demands, more emphasis should be given to the use of milk and its products, particularly lower-fat varieties, in the teenage diet (see Q2.5). Three 200 ml (7 fl oz) glasses of milk a day and either 45 g (1.5 oz) of cheese or 125 ml (around 5 fl oz) of yoghurt would together meet their daily requirements. Both nutrition and physical activity are important for the formation of strong healthy bones and the prevention of osteoporosis in later life.

Q3.68 What guidance exists on school meals?

The provision of food at school, especially for older children, is usually in the form of a cash-cafeteria service (see Q3.61). A DHSS survey (1989) showed that older children, especially girls who were eating out of school in take-away cafés or fast food outlets, were selecting foods of rather lower nutrient density than those consuming school meals. They had a lower intake of many nutrients, especially iron but also calcium and vitamin A. There is little to suggest that things have changed during the intervening period. As described in Q3.63, regulations and guidance for nutritional standards for school lunches were published by the Government in 2000. These regulations require schools to provide meals that comply with quantifiable nutritional standards. However, given the choice available in secondary school cafeterias, the challenge will be to guide pupils to make appropriate choices.

Q3.69 What problems do nurses and other health professionals face when trying to improve the nutritional knowledge of children?

Teenagers may not be receptive to efforts to change their behaviour, not least because growing independence may make them hostile to intervention by health professionals, as well as by teachers and parents. They are also unlikely to be motivated by information about risk of increased disease in later life. Where nutritional concerns are expressed by teenagers, they tend to be in relation to how diet may lower weight and improve shape, or to worries about environmental issues. This age group is very susceptible to peer group pressure. These factors must be taken into account when trying to develop methods to improve the nutritional knowledge of adolescents.

Q3.70 Are there special considerations for pregnant teenagers?

The UK has the highest rate of teenage pregnancy in Europe: 56,000 babies are born to girls aged 15–19 years each year (The Social Exclusion Unit 1999). Pregnant teenagers, particularly those who may still be in their own growth phase, do have increased needs for nutrients in pregnancy. Although most growth occurs before menarche, linear growth is not usually completed until approximately 4 years later. The diet of the pregnant teenager must therefore meet the requirement for their own growth and development, along with the extra demands of the growing fetus. Nutrient requirements may also remain relatively high in pregnant teenagers who have completed the growth phase because stores are likely to be low in women who have recently experienced rapid growth.

Teenage pregnancy involves increased risk of mortality and morbidity for both the mother and the infant (Ranjan, 1993). A higher incidence of maternal bleeding, difficult labour and delivery, anaemia and hypertensive complications has been reported among teenagers (National Dairy Council, 1989). Maternal mortality is 2.5 times greater in 15-year-old girls than in 20- to 24-year-old women (Rees and Mahan, 1988). The infants of teenage mothers are more likely to have a low birthweight, which increases the risk of death and illness, particularly throughout the perinatal period. Although the increased prevalence of low-birthweight infants among teenagers has been linked with socioeconomic and behavioural factors (smoking, alcohol consumption, drug use), inadequate weight gain during pregnancy is also a key factor. Young adolescents (less than 2 years post-menarche) may deliver smaller infants for a given maternal weight gain than older women. It is therefore essential that the diet provides adequate protein and energy throughout pregnancy.

The demands for calcium are also relatively high because of continuing consolidation of the mother's skeleton and the calcification of the fetal skeleton and teeth. Iron, zinc and folic acid are also key nutrients because they are involved in the growth of new tissue. Dietary habits are often more erratic among pregnant teenagers than pregnant adults. Low intakes and blood levels of several nutrients have been reported, including vitamin A, vitamin C, folic acid, calcium, iron and zinc (Stevens-Simon and McAnarney, 1988). The importance of deriving energy from foods of high nutrient density, such as milk and dairy products, lean meat, fish, cereals, fruit and vegetables, should be emphasised. Although most teenage pregnancies are unplanned, all adult women and older girls should be made aware of the need for folic acid supplementation, before and up to week 12 of pregnancy (see Q3.2). This is essential to reduce the risk of neural tube defects. The need for further vitamin supplementation should be advised on an individual basis. Pregnant teenagers can be a difficult group to reach to provide relevant dietary advice. They may face considerable financial problems, with the amount of money available to spend on food being very limited. Knowledge of both food and food preparation may also be poor. The provision of dietary advice on how to select good food on a low income may be vital to the health of the teenage mother and the growing child (see Q3.105)

Q3.71 Is constant snacking ('grazing') bad for growing children?

Concern is sometimes expressed over the increase in consumption of 'junk food' and high-fat and sugar snacks among teenagers. As teenagers tend to start eating away from home more, they have the luxury of making their own choices for the first time, and are notorious for snacking and missing out on important meals such as breakfast. The term 'grazing' has been adopted to describe the constant eating of snack foods as opposed to conventional meals. A study in 1985 among 15–25 year olds found that 58% eat breakfast daily,

33% eat a cooked lunch and 78% consume a cooked evening meal
(Bull, 1985). Skipping meals, particularly breakfast, is more likely
among adolescents than among younger children. This can make
teenagers feel lethargic and lack concentration. A light breakfast of
low-fat yoghurt and fresh fruit, or cereal and fruit juice, is much
better than no food at all.

Teenagers and young adults are more likely than adults to have
an eating pattern based on convenience foods such as chips, sauces,
soft drinks, nuts, cheese, rice and pasta, savoury pies and cooked
meat dishes (Barker et al., 1990). Although 'fast foods' such as
hamburgers and chips may provide protein and some vitamins and
minerals, they are generally low in vitamin A and fibre and do not
contain much vitamin C or calcium. Some 'fast foods' are also high
in sodium, fat and calories (energy). It is therefore important to
encourage parents to provide a variety of healthy foods at home,
especially fruit, vegetables, fish, wholegrain cereals and pulses such
as beans, peas and lentils. Frequent consumption of snacks need not
be detrimental to health if they are of high nutrient density. Healthy
snacks include fruit, vegetables, sandwiches, low-fat milk products
and breakfast cereal.

> Q3.72 Many teenagers are adopting a vegetarian style of eating. Are there
> associated problems?

Adolescence is a period of developing social awareness, which may be
reflected in a desire to adopt vegetarian, vegan or 'health food' regimens (see Q4.18). Women are more likely to be non-meat eating than
men, particularly in the 16–24 year age group (Realeat, 1993). Around
10% of adolescent girls aged 15–18 years currently describe themselves
as vegetarian or vegan (Gregory et al., 2000). This is not in itself a problem and can be a healthy way of eating. However, maintaining a good
nutritional status on a vegan diet (no foods of animal origin) can be
more difficult, particularly for teenagers who have very high requirements for calcium, iron and zinc. The unsupervised adoption of vegan
diets can lead to problems among teenagers who have increased
requirements for several nutrients, especially at the time of the growth
spurt. Those adopting a vegan diet during the growth period may have
difficulty meeting their energy needs because of the high bulk of the
diet. Such diets may also be low in fat and therefore in energy. If the

amount of energy provided by the diet is insufficient, the body will use protein as an energy source, rendering this protein unavailable for tissue synthesis and growth. Deficiencies of iron, calcium, zinc, vitamin B_{12} and protein can also result. A planned vegetarian diet, consisting of a wide variety of foods, can provide all the essential nutrients and there is no reason why teenagers cannot thrive on a well-balanced vegetarian diet based around wholemeal bread, pasta, potatoes and rice, eaten with a wide variety of vegetables, fruit, nuts and seeds. Nurses should offer advice and support to teenagers wishing to adopt such diets and help them to obtain reliable information. Children who become vegan and cut out all dairy products and eggs may need to take supplements of vitamin B_{12}, or eat fortified breakfast cereals served with calcium-fortified soya milk (or fruit juice) (see Q2.16 and Q2.37).

Q3.73 Do children who are keen on sport have special dietary needs?

Teenagers who participate regularly in sport are likely to have an increased energy requirement. An adequate intake of water, protein, iron and the B vitamins is also essential. These increased needs can, however, be met through a balanced diet.

Intensive training at critical stages in adolescence may interfere with growth and development. Although boys more frequently participate in competitive sport than girls, most research has focused on the effects of intensive training on the timing of the onset of puberty in females. Some highly trained female athletes, such as gymnasts and ballet dancers, may display late onset of menstruation or develop amenorrhoea. This has been linked to osteoporosis in later life (Cann et al., 1984). This delay in menarche has been attributed to a lack of body fat relative to lean body mass, but the interaction between exercise, reproductive function and the body fat:lean body mass ratio remains unclear. Teenage athletes may also be at risk of iron deficiency caused by red blood cell destruction, increased need for red blood cell and tissue synthesis during puberty or poor dietary intake (see British Nutrition Foundation 2001b).

Q3.74 How common are eating disorders and what advice can be offered to
        parents?

In recent years, there has been increasing concern that the pressure to conform to a 'slim image' and 'to diet' is resulting in a rise in the prevalence of eating disorders. These range from anorexia nervosa, which is essentially a condition of self-starvation, to bulimia nervosa, characterised by recurrent episodes of binge eating. In 1992, the Royal College of Psychiatrists estimated that around 60 000 people are known to clinics as having anorexia or bulimia nervosa in the UK. However, the Eating Disorders Association currently believe the number to be nearer to 90 000 and many more are likely to have undiagnosed eating disorders. The illness is more common among women (90% of cases), particularly young women between the ages of 15 and 25 years. Studies have documented an increase in dietary restraint and dieting, particularly among adolescent girls, e.g. the Young Person's Health Survey (Department of Health, 1998d) found that 47% of girls aged 16–19 try to lose weight. Although the incidence is much lower, eating disorders can occur in boys, particularly during adolescence.

Eating disorders commonly last for 6 years but can persist throughout life, with many people fluctuating between anorexia and bulimia nervosa (Eating Disorders Association, 1995). Anorexia nervosa is characterised by a profound self-induced starvation, marked weight loss, cessation of menstrual periods in women, a distorted body image and a fear of fatness. Many people with anorexia exercise vigorously or use slimming pills to keep their weight as low as possible. Slimmers are at increased risk of calcium, iron, vitamin A, riboflavin and vitamin B_6 deficiency. Prolonged anorexia can lead to depression, disturbed sleep, general weakness, and a range of health complications such as heart, kidney and gastrointestinal, and fertility problems. Women who have had anorexia are at risk of osteoporosis. Anorexia also has one of the highest mortality rates for any psychiatric condition, estimated to be around 13–20% per annum (Howlett et al., 1995).

Bulimia nervosa is characterised by constant dieting with episodes of binge eating, followed by purging, with self-induced vomiting, laxative abuse or both. Sufferers are often overweight as children and become bulimic in their late teens and early 20s. Long-term consequences include muscle weakness, an irregular heart beat, epileptic fits and kidney damage. Regular vomiting can also cause the tooth enamel to dissolve.

People with anorexia and bulimia should be encouraged to seek medical advice as soon as possible. The treatment for both of these disorders will involve psychiatric input. It is important that the promotion of good nutrition among teenagers does not enhance the culture of weight loss and increase the number of young people at risk of these serious illnesses. Although an awareness of sensible eating and the avoidance of being overweight are important for children and adolescents, this must be carefully controlled both in the school and in the home environment. Maintenance of a healthy weight should focus on an increase in physical activity, rather than dietary restraint.

For more information on eating disorders, the reader is referred to Cieslik et al. (1999).

Q3.75 Could teenagers who are taking drugs or alcohol be at risk nutritionally?

Many drugs have known adverse interactions with nutrients, increasing the risk of deficiencies. The most common drug to reduce the absorption of several nutrients is alcohol. There is concern about the increase in alcohol consumption among teenagers in the UK. The Health of Young People survey (Department of Health, 1998d) found that 26% of boys consume over 10 units per week and 23% of girls drink more than 7 units per week by the age of 16. By the age of 18, these figures rose to 54% and 45%, respectively. Nutrient interactions with alcohol are complex but it may alter the absorption and metabolism of many nutrients, including amino acids, calcium and vitamins such as thiamin (vitamin B_1), folic acid and vitamin C (see Chapter 2). It can increase the requirement for some vitamins and it is generally accepted that regular drinkers are likely to have poorer diets than non-drinkers. A high alcohol consumption may therefore threaten an adequate nutritional intake, particularly among adolescent girls who are dieting. In addition, smoking and alcohol drinking tend to go hand in hand.

Q3.76 Is vitamin C status reduced in teenagers who smoke?

Teenage smoking appears to be increasing in the UK and can adversely affect nutritional status. In the Health of Young People survey (Department of Health, 1998d), 49% of boys and 54% of girls claimed to have smoked cigarettes by the age of 15; 13% of boys and 14% of girls aged 15 were regular smokers. Tobacco components appear to influence the metabolism and possibly also the absorption of vitamin C, making it likely that smokers have a higher requirement for this vitamin. This may be of particular concern among teenage girls who are slimming and restricting their dietary intake or in those taking oral contraceptives, which may further reduce blood vitamin C levels (Rivers, 1975). Calcium metabolism can also be influenced adversely by smoking. Smoking may indirectly affect nutritional intake by reducing the amount of money available to teenagers to spend on food.

Nutrition and Women of Child-bearing Age

Q3.77 Premenstrual syndrome is a problem many women have to live with. Can diet help?

A number of symptoms have been described in premenstrual syndrome (PMS), including water retention, irritability, depression, backache and breast tenderness. These usually disappear soon after menstruation begins. A variety of dietary factors has been suggested to play a role, including several vitamins and minerals and essential fatty acids (Stewart et al., 1992). Vitamin B_6 has been promoted widely by the media as a self-help approach to PMS. This is discussed more fully in Q5.4.

Q3.78. It has been suggested that, if pregnancies are too frequent, a woman's nutrient stores do not become adequately replenished between pregnancies. Is this true and can dietary change help?

Nutritional status at the time of conception is an important determinant of embryonic and fetal growth (see Q3.1). Women who are underweight at the time of conception are at greater risk of having a low-birthweight baby. Low preconceptional vitamin intake has also been linked with the development of neural tube defects and other fetal abnormalities. Very short intervals between pregnancies may not allow a woman's stores to be adequately replenished. Women must therefore be encouraged to continue to eat a varied and adequate diet beyond pregnancy and lactation to ensure that there are no nutritional imbalances. It is the nurse's role to advise individual patients as to whether the use of supplements may be useful to ensure adequacy in cases of closely spaced births.

Q3.79 Do healthy women need to consider dietary supplements

There are times when the requirement for certain vitamins and minerals may be increased and the use of dietary supplements may be useful (see Q2.37). Women with high menstrual losses and/or iron-deficiency anaemia will benefit from iron supplements. Pregnant women and breast-feeding mothers may require vitamin D supplements to achieve intakes of 10 μg/day. The recommended intake of an extra 400 μg/day of folic acid for women planning a baby and during the first 12 weeks of pregnancy is easily met using a supplement. The need for calcium supplementation in women with osteoporosis is still being debated, but may be useful in women who find it difficult to increase their calcium intake. Elderly or housebound women, and those who cover up most of their skin, may need a vitamin D supplement of 10 μg/day. Supplements can also be useful during recovery from an illness. However, a healthy balanced diet should provide sufficient amounts of all the necessary vitamins and minerals required by the body and supplements should not be used as an excuse to eat a poor diet.

Q3.80 How common is iron-deficiency anaemia and how can it be avoided?

Women of reproductive age are at risk of iron deficiency as a result of menstrual losses or during pregnancy and lactation, when the demands for iron are increased substantially. The use of intrauterine contraceptive devices (IUDs) may increase the risk of anaemia as a result of increased menstrual blood loss. The avoidance of iron-rich foods during dieting can also lead to deficiency. Adolescent girls, who have high iron requirements for growth, are especially vulnerable.

Even though iron requirements are not as high in post-menopausal women, it is still important to include a range of iron-containing foods in the diet. The best-absorbed sources of iron are animal products such as meat, fish and poultry (see Q2.6).

Q3.81 How common is obesity and how best can it be tackled?

Obesity has more than doubled in the UK since 1980 and well over half the population is now overweight or obese. A larger number of women than men are obese (20% and 17%, respectively, in England) (British Nutrition Foundation, 1999a). Obesity is not merely a cosmetic or social problem because it is linked to a number of diseases, including cancer and heart disease (see Q4.6). Despite studies confirming a strong genetic influence on obesity, it is now accepted that obesity can occur only when the energy equation is unbalanced, i.e. when energy intake exceeds energy expenditure (see Q4.7).

Pregnancy can be a critical period for the development of future obesity in some women. Excessive weight and fat gain in pregnancy can place the mother at risk of being overweight or obese postpartum. Body weight and fatness may increase with each successive pregnancy if the retained weight is not lost between reproductive cycles. Some women, however, gain weight after the birth of the baby, suggesting that lactation, diet and activity related to child rearing might be important, as well as child-bearing. The prevalence of obesity in men and women increases greatly during adulthood and peaks in late middle age. There is little evidence that the menopause represents a risk period for extra weight gain, but loss of oestrogen activity has been linked to increased central obesity.

Environmental changes, including a more sedentary lifestyle and the ready availability of energy-dense foods, are the most likely factors to explain the rapid increase in the prevalence of obesity. Education about the importance of a low-fat diet and an increase in physical activity is therefore the key strategy to improved weight loss (see Q4.8–4.12).

Q3.82 What is the best advice for women who have only a few pounds to lose?

For those wishing to lose a few pounds, being more physically active is the key. Taking opportunistic physical activity, such as walking short distances instead of taking the car or opting for the stairs instead of a lift, may be all that is needed (see Q3.87).

Q3.83 Is it true that fat deposited around the waist is a more serious problem than fat on the hips and thighs?

Both women and men with a high proportion of abdominal fat (central obesity) are at greater risk of heart disease. The distribution of fat is generally considered a better predictor of cardiovascular risk than body mass index (see Q4.4). Central obesity is associated with unfavourable metabolic disturbances such as reduced insulin sensitivity and glucose intolerance. Fat distribution is measured as the waist: hip ratio, a high ratio being associated with elevated cardiovascular risk. Women tend to have lower waist:hip ratios than men, but the ratio often increases after the menopause when there is both an increase in total fat mass and in the amount of fat deposited in the upper body. This change in fat distribution may contribute to the greater risk of coronary heart disease seen in women after the menopause.

A simple waist measurement can be a quick predictor. A waist measurement in women of over 80 cm (32 inches) is associated with increased risk to health, with 88 cm (35 inches) associated with substantial risk to health.

Q3.84   With regard to heart disease prevention, what is the most appropriate advice for women?

At all ages women are at lower risk from coronary heart disease (CHD) than men. In premenopausal women, this has been attributed to the protective effect of the hormone oestrogen. Although the risk of CHD increases for women after the menopause, it remains below that of men despite the prevalence of recognised risk factors. Most studies on risk factors for heart disease have been performed in men and there is a need to extend these studies to women. However, there is a limited amount of research to suggest that women can tolerate some of the risk factors better than men. The protective effect of high-density lipoprotein (HDL) cholesterol appears to be stronger in women and, at any given level of blood cholesterol, the risk of heart disease is lower than in men. This has led to considerable discussion about whether attempts to lower blood lipid levels in women will produce the same benefits as in men. It has been argued that encouraging a low-fat diet in women may not lower CHD risk substantially and may have adverse effects on the balance of the diet in terms of calcium and iron intake (Crouse, 1989). The general recommendations on smoking, physical activity, being overweight and the general benefit of a healthy diet, however, remain the same.

Q3.85   What is the advice for women about alcohol intake?

Heavy alcohol consumption increases the risk of cardiovascular disease, some forms of cancer (e.g. mouth, pharynx, oesophagus, liver, breast), stroke, cirrhosis, accidents and suicide. However, drinking moderately (1–2 units/day) may provide some protection against heart disease, particularly in postmenopausal women and men aged over 40 years (Department of Health, 1995a). Although wine in particular has been advocated as beneficial in moderate quantities, as yet this remains speculative. Wine drinkers tend to be more healthy because of a number of lifestyle characteristics, e.g. they are often of higher social class. Amid much controversy, the Department of Health recommendations for alcohol intake were raised to 3–4 units/day in men and 2–3 units/day in women (Department of Health, 1995a). Lower amounts are advised for women because they usually weigh less than men and metabolise alcohol differently, and are less tolerant to the adverse effects of alcohol.

Drinking heavily throughout pregnancy (more than 80 g/day) is linked with fetal alcohol syndrome which is characterised by reduced birthweight and length, and a variety of congenital abnormalities (Ernhart et al., 1987; Abel, 1998) (see Q3.6). Affected children are at increased risk of learning disabilities and stunted growth. Although there is little evidence that drinking less than 80 g of alcohol per week (equivalent to a bottle of wine) is harmful to the fetus, alcohol consumption can reduce birthweight. It is therefore recommended that women avoid alcohol during pregnancy.

A British Nutrition Foundation Briefing Paper on the subject of alcohol is being prepared and will be available towards the end of 2001.

Q3.86 Can thrush be related to food intake?

Candida albicans is a strain of yeast present in almost every human body, the growth of which is kept under control by the immune system. However if the immune system is suppressed *C. albicans* can grow in the mucous membranes such as the mouth, throat, vulva and vagina, causing a condition known as candidiasis or thrush. Candidiasis is a common infection. Almost three-quarters of all women will experience at least one episode in their lifetime. Candidiasis may also affect people taking antibiotics. As the antibiotic temporarily kills some of the harmless but important bacteria that inhabit the body, this provides an opportunity for *C. albicans* to take hold. People with diabetes have thrush more frequently than the general population. This may be a result of the elevated glucose blood level. Pregnancy may cause the condition and some experts believe that oral contraceptives are also implicated. Both result in hormonal changes, which may alter the vaginal environment and promote the proliferation of the fungus. Immunosuppressed and AIDS patients also contract it readily. Candidiasis will affect individuals differently. One may have gastrointestinal disorders, while another may have respiratory problems and still another may have dermatological manifestations (skin rash). 'Live' yoghurt, eaten or applied to the affected area, may help to prevent recurrent candidiasis. This is because live yoghurt contains useful bacteria that stop candida organisms growing. Alternatively, multi-acidophilus powder can be taken as a dietary supplement and this has the same effect as live yoghurt. Some complementary therapists recommend avoiding sweet food, white flour and starchy foods, alleging that this deprives the *C. albicans* of nutrients. This approach is not, however, supported by sufficient evidence and can potentially lead to nutritional imbalances if foods are excluded without appropriate dietary advice.

Q3.87 What are the recommendations for physical activity?

Thirty minutes of moderate activity on at least 5 days of the week is recommended to reduce the risk of several diseases, including strokes and heart attacks (Department of Health, 1995b). Other benefits include aiding weight loss, reducing stress and maintaining well-being. However, the activity levels of adults in the UK fall far below this recommendation and evidence suggests that women in the UK are even less active than men. An increasing reliance on cars and labour-saving devices in the home and on sedentary amusements such as television watching has led to a decline in everyday activity. Appropriate campaigns are required to motivate women and encourage them to be more physically active (see Q4.10).

Nutrition and Men

Q3.88 Are there any particular nutritional issues that need to be addressed?

The major cause of death among men in the UK is cardiovascular disease, accounting for 41% of all deaths in men under 75 years in 1996. Coronary heart disease alone accounts for 28% of premature deaths in men, totalling 81 000 deaths in 1996 (British Heart Foundation, 1998). The most common risk factors for heart disease among men include smoking, a lack of physical activity and a poor diet. The most common forms of cancer among men are lung, colorectal and prostate cancers. There is evidence that there is a dietary component in the aetiology of each of these (Department of Health, 1998c). Although the incidence of lung cancer has fallen over the last 20 years as smoking rates have declined, the numbers of men developing testicular and prostate cancer have risen. Men often pay less attention to their health than women and are less likely to use primary healthcare services. Healthy eating and lifestyle messages need to be more specifically targeted at men, in the same way that women's lifestyle magazines have done for many years.

Q3.89 Do healthy men need to consider dietary supplements?

Men who consume a healthy balanced diet (see Q1.8) should obtain all the nutrients required. Men who are consuming restricted diets such as low-calorie (energy) or vegan diets may benefit from using dietary supplements. Supplements may also be useful during recovery from illness.

Q3.90 How common is obesity and how best can it be tackled?

The prevalence of obesity has more than doubled in the UK over the last 20 years, increasing from 6% in men in 1980 to 17% in 1997 and from 8% to 20% in women over the same time period (see Q3.81 and Q4.5). Although, in the UK, the prevalence of obesity has been reported to be higher in the manual classes than in the non-manual classes, in men the relationship is less consistent than in women. A low educational attainment has, however, been linked to obesity in both sexes (see British Nutrition Foundation, 1999a).

The health consequences of obesity are several and varied, ranging from an increased risk of premature death to non-fatal but debilitating illnesses (see Q4.6).

Obesity can occur only when energy intake remains higher than energy expenditure for an extended period of time. The rising prevalence of obesity can best be tackled by providing education about the need for positive lifestyle changes at both the individual and the population level. Dietary strategies form an important part of the treatment of obesity, but long-term strategies that deal with both diet and activity should be promoted (see Q4.8–4.12).

Q3.91 What is the best advice for men who have only a few pounds to lose?

For men wishing to lose a few pounds, incorporating more physical activity into everyday life or at work, by changing habits a little, may be all that is needed. Examples include using the stairs instead of the lift or getting off the bus a stop early and walking the rest of the way.

Q3.92 Is it true that fat deposited around the waist is a more serious problem than fat on the hips and thighs?

The accumulation of fat around the waist, rather than the hips and thighs, is referred to as central obesity. This can be defined according to the waist:hip ratio or more simply by measuring waist circumference. In men a waist:hip ratio above 1.0 or a waist circumference over 94 cm (37 inches) is associated with an increased risk to health. A waist circumference above 102 cm (40 inches) confers a substantial risk to health.

Q3.93 With regard to heart disease prevention, what is the most appropriate advice for men?

Men have a greater risk of CHD than women. Despite the fall in death rates from CHD that has occurred since 1970 in both sexes and all age groups in the UK, heart disease remains the most common single cause of premature death in middle-aged men (British Heart Foundation, 1998). A large number of risk factors for the disease have been identified. Cigarette smoking is a very important risk factor but several aspects of the diet have also been implicated. Obesity predisposes to the development of hypertension and diabetes, both of which are very strong risk factors for CHD. Maintaining a healthy body weight is therefore a very important factor in the prevention of heart disease.

High intakes of fat, particularly saturated fatty acids, from spreads, fatty meat, biscuits, cakes, snack foods and dairy products, increase blood levels of low-density lipoprotein (LDL) cholesterol (see Q2.3, Q2.4 and Table 2.1). Choosing lean cuts of meat, reduced fat spreads and low-fat dairy products will reduce the intake of these fatty acids. Polyunsaturated fatty acids of the *n*-6 family (rich sources include sunflower oil and corn oil) and monounsaturated fatty acids (rich sources include olive oil and rapeseed oil) can lower LDL-cholesterol levels (see Q4.2). Soluble fibre, which is found in oats, legumes and vegetables, can also lower blood cholesterol levels. The type of polyunsaturated fatty acids found in oil-rich fish (*n*-3 or ω-3) do not lower cholesterol, but they do have beneficial effects on other blood fats (see below).

A diet rich in fruit and vegetables will provide a range of antioxidant nutrients, including vitamin E, vitamin C and β-carotene. Such a diet is thought to protect against oxidative damage in the body, which in turn is thought to be an important factor in the development of heart disease and cancer (see British Nutrition Foundation, 1992; see Q4.2).

The consumption of at least one portion of oil-rich fish per week (e.g. mackerel, salmon or herring) has also been recommended to reduce the risk of CHD. The *n*-3 fatty acids found in fish can reduce triglyceride levels in the blood, beneficially influence heart arrhythmias and also help to prevent blood clots from forming (see British Nutrition Foundation, 1999c).

Other dietary factors linked to heart disease include a high salt intake and heavy drinking, which have both been implicated in the development of hypertension (see Q2.28 and Q4.2).

Q3.94 What is the advice on alcohol intake for men?

Moderate alcohol consumption (around two drinks per day) is associated with a reduced risk of CHD (Kannel and Ellison, 1996). At levels of intake above this, the risk of CVD (CHD and stroke) begins to increase. Current advice for men is to consume no more than 3–4 units of alcohol per day (a maximum of 28 units per week) (Department of Health, 1995a). An intake at this level is not associated with any significant health risk. However, 28% of men in Britain have an alcohol intake above this recommended limit (British Heart Foundation, 1998). Age and geographical region affect alcohol consumption; intake is higher in the younger age groups and in the north of England. However, in men, alcohol consumption does not vary with socioeconomic status.

Q3.95 Are there any substantiated links between diet and cancer?

The incidence of several types of cancer has been linked to a number of dietary and nutritional factors and poor diet has been estimated to account for about a quarter of all cancer deaths in this country (Department of Health, 1999). Dietary recommendations have been produced by the Department of Health and the World Cancer Research Fund (World Cancer Research Fund, 1997; Department of Health, 1998c). Studies have shown an association between fruit and vegetable consumption and colorectal and stomach cancer, and a low intake of these foods has been implicated in several other cancers. For this reason, the consumption of at least five portions of fruit and vegetables every day is recommended. There is some evidence of a link between consumption of red and processed meat and colorectal cancer (Department of Health, 1998c). A reduction in meat consumption may, however, have adverse nutritional implications; in particular, iron intake may be reduced. For this reason, it is recommended that the current average intake of red and processed meat (about 90 g/day cooked weight, or 8–10 portions a week) should not rise. There is also some evidence to suggest that a diet rich in non-starch polysaccharides (fibre) may help protect against colorectal and pancreatic cancer, and adults in the UK are advised to increase their intake to 18 g/day (see Q2.1 and Q4.3).

Q3.96 We are all encouraged to be more active these days. Does active participation in sport necessitate a different type of diet or special supplements?

Regular activity confers health benefits which can prolong and promote well-being. Active participation in sport does not necessitate a different type of diet. A balanced diet, supplying adequate energy, should provide all the nutrients required. Supplementing a balanced diet with vitamins and minerals has not been shown to increase physical performance. The emphasis in a sportsperson's diet is placed on increasing the proportion of carbohydrate foods to meet the increased demands for energy. During high-exercise intensity, the body uses glucose, from its glycogen stores in the muscle, as the main source of fuel. A diet containing plenty of foods rich in carbohydrate (see Q1.6) and low in fat will maximise the carbohydrate stores and sustain strenuous activity for more prolonged periods of time. Recreational exercisers who wish to improve their performance may benefit from increasing their carbohydrate intake on the day of taking exercise. When the body sweats it loses water; drinking plenty of water is essential, particularly during prolonged exercise and as an aid to recovery after exertion. For more information on nutrition and sport, see the British Nutrition Foundation Briefing Paper (2001b)

Nutrition and the Menopause

Q3.97 Are there any nutritional issues that need to be addressed at this time?

During the menopause, as with any other time in life, it is important to aim for a varied and well-balanced diet (see Q1.7 and Q1.8). There are also some specific nutritional issues that may be of interest. Intake of calcium and vitamin D is important, along with physical activity, to ensure optimal bone health (see Q2.5 and Q2.22). Iron requirements change when menstruation stops. Also, there has recently been an interest in phyto-oestrogens and their possible role in alleviating symptoms associated with the menopause, such as hot flushes (Cassidy et al., 1994). These substances are found in vegetables and pulses; soya beans are the richest source (see Q5.10).

For those watching their weight, the dietary messages are the same. The aim should be to cut down a little more on the amount of food eaten and, in particular, care should be taken to ensure that intakes of fat and alcohol are not excessive – these are concentrated sources of calories. There are no miracle cures for weight loss; sensible eating and gentle regular exercise are by far the best long-term solutions to the problem.

Q3.98 What are the risk factors for osteoporosis at the time of the menopause?

Bone health can be influenced by a number of factors. There may be genetic influences, e.g. African-Caribbean groups tend to have larger and heavier bones than white or Asian populations. Nutritional influences are also important. Calcium and vitamin D are the nutrients considered most important in relation to bone health, but other nutrients are also of significance, e.g. vitamin K (Buttriss et al., 2000) and various other minerals. Smoking has been suggested as a possible factor associated with increased risk of osteoporosis, and alcohol has been found to reduce bone mineral density (Department of Health, 1998a). A high sodium intake increases urinary excretion of calcium, although there is some evidence that this is counteracted by an increase in absorption (Department of Health, 1998a).

It is well established that bone loss accelerates in the years immediately after the menopause. The role of calcium in the prevention of bone mineral loss during the menopause has been studied extensively. Calcium supplementation does not seem to have any major effect on bone mineral density at the time of the menopause, perhaps because any effects are masked by other changes going on at this time. However, studies on women 5 years postmenopause are more positive and show a slower loss of bone with calcium supplementation (Department of Health, 1998a). Body levels of vitamin D are also known to be important, because both nutrients are needed for a strong skeleton (see Q2.22).

However, it is now being recognised that calcium and vitamin D are not the only nutrients to be considered, e.g. there is now considerable interest in vitamin K (see Q2.23). Advice should focus on the importance of a varied and balanced diet. With regard to calcium, some of the best sources are dairy products, including milk, cheese, yoghurts and dairy-based desserts. Other sources include canned fish eaten with bones, bread and cereal foods made from fortified flour, pulses, some green vegetables, e.g. broccoli (spinach is a poor source as the calcium is unavailable for absorption), tofu, and some nuts and seeds, e.g. sesame seeds and peanuts.

Physical activity is another important part of the equation (see Q3.87 and Q4.10). This does not have to mean high level aerobics (although those who enjoy this sort of activity should go ahead), but can simply involve brisk walking, gardening or swimming. Weight-bearing exercise is of particular benefit at this time of life, e.g. jogging, brisk walking and, in particular, weight training. This can help to maintain bone strength.

Advice to avoid smoking and to drink within sensible limits is also important. For further information on osteoporosis, see Q4.15.

Q3.99 Are phyto-oestrogens an alternative to HRT?

There has been recent debate about the role of phyto-oestrogens in helping to alleviate the symptoms of the menopause (Cassidy et al., 1994) (see Q5.10). Phyto-oestrogens are a family of oestrogenic plant-derived substances found mainly in soya beans and soya products, although they are also present in red clover and chick peas (and in other pulses and vegetables in lower concentrations). The amount of phyto-oestrogens needed to exert an effect in humans is suggested to be 30–50 mg/day; this is achievable by consuming a diet high in soya beans and soya products.

Some studies have shown that phyto-oestrogens can alleviate some of the symptoms of the menopause, such as hot flushes and vaginitis (Albertazzi et al., 1999). Other studies, however, have shown no effect. At the present time, phyto-oestrogens should not be viewed as an alternative to hormone replacement therapy (HRT). Further trials in progress in this area may yield more conclusive results.

Ethnic Minority Groups

Q3.100 What advice should be given to ethnic minority groups in terms of their traditional diets, particularly in relation to weaning?

Many aspects of the traditional diets of ethnic minority groups are beneficial and, in health terms, the Westernisation of these diets may be disadvantageous. Although the older generation of immigrants often wishes to maintain traditional eating patterns, diets among the younger generation are changing and as a result contain more sugar, fat, processed foods and take-aways. Concern has been raised about the nutritional adequacy of diets that combine traditional and Western eating habits or adopt modifications of Western eating patterns (e.g. the inclusion of a lot of milk and sweet foods but rejection of savoury items). In particular, such diets may not be adequate to provide for the needs of young infants. Weight faltering is considered by most health professionals to be more common, particularly among Asian children. Children from families of several ethnic minority groups are more likely to experience problems around the time of weaning (Department of Health, 1994c).

Both the choice of weaning food and the time that weaning is initiated depend on religious and cultural factors. Some infants from Asian and Chinese minority groups receive large amounts of infant formula or cows' milk as their primary source of nutrition for an inappropriately long time. Beyond 6 months, these foods are not able to support the requirements of the growing child. In particular, iron-deficiency anaemia (see Q3.44) is more common among Asian children than Europid children living in the same areas, which can be exacerbated by use of cows' milk as the main drink because it is low in iron when compared with formula.

Prolonged bottle-feeding and the consumption of large volumes of fluid (possibly of relatively low nutrient density) can reduce appetite at meal times, resulting in both a poorer nutrient intake and delayed progress to a mixed diet (see Q3.43). Among Asian families sugar and honey are more commonly added to bottle feeds – a practice that has been associated with a higher prevalence of dental caries (see Q3.47).

Hindu parents often wean their children onto vegetarian diets. Less restrictive lactovegetarian or lacto-ovovegetarian diets can adequately provide for the child's nutritional needs, although most convenience weaning foods contain both meat and vegetables. Vegan diets, however, are often lower in nutrients such as vitamin D, iron and vitamin B_{12} (see Q4.20 and Q4.21). Weaning practices in African-Caribbean infants have not been published in detail, but cornmeal and banana are usually introduced early, with other traditional foods provided later in infancy (such as plantains, sweet potatoes and yams). These foods have a low density and a relatively low protein:energy ratio. They also tend to be bulky, so that children may not be able to consume an amount sufficient to meet their needs. Where there is any doubt about the adequacy of energy intake, parents should be advised to supplement the diet with an appropriate source of fat, although care must be taken to ensure that the protein content is adequate to meet the needs of the growing child. High levels of phytate and other inhibitors can reduce the intake of several micronutrients, especially iron and zinc. Vegetarian diets should contain larger amounts of vitamin C to enhance iron absorption. Where there is likely to be micronutrient deficiencies, a multivitamin and mineral supplement could be recommended.

There are several other difficulties, particularly for new immigrants, that can affect the young child during weaning. New mothers may feel isolated and deprived of support from their wider community network of family and friends. They may not speak English or know where they can obtain advice. The foods on sale may be unfamiliar and traditional foods very difficult to find. Where dietary change is to be recommended, advice must be tailored to the person's customary eating pattern. To achieve this, health professionals need to acquire a knowledge and understanding of the client's diet, religious beliefs, cultural habits, lifestyle and attitudes. It is important that clients are asked about their food choices rather than assumptions being made, e.g. it cannot be assumed that all Hindus are vegetarian or that all Muslims avoid alcohol.

Q3.101 What about vitamin D intake?

The darker skin of Asian women reduces the access of UV light to the structures in the skin that synthesise vitamin D. Also, dietary intake of vitamin D may be poor, particularly for those with vegan diets (see Q3.16). This is also a problem for Asian infants and children (Department of Health, 1994c; Gregory et al., 2000). Rickets caused by simple vitamin D deficiency is more common among Asian children but, as in European children, is declining. Vitamin supplements for pregnant women and children under 5 years, dietary education and appropriate advice to increase the exposure of the skin to sunlight can improve vitamin D status. Asian women who choose to cover their skin when outdoors or spend little time outdoors may also benefit from specific advice on vitamin D (see Q2.22).

Q3.102 Are there ethnic differences in the prevalence of obesity and diabetes?

The prevalence and incidence of type 2 or non-insulin-dependent diabetes mellitus (NIDDM) are higher in several ethnic minority populations in the UK, e.g. the prevalence of diabetes in Asians in Britain has been shown to be some four times higher than that in Europeans (Mather and Keen, 1985; McKeigue et al., 1991). Gestational diabetes (appearing in pregnancy) is also more common among Asian women. The influence of obesity on type 2 diabetes in this population is unclear. The mean body mass index (BMI) of Asian and Europid men with diabetes has been shown to be similar, although Asian women with diabetes often have a higher BMI than their Europid counterparts (Nicholl et al., 1986). Type 2 diabetes, however, remains more prevalent among South Asians compared with Europeans, in all groupings of BMI, but this measure of obesity may be an unreliable guide when comparing different ethnic groups because of differences in body fat distribution. South Asians tend to accumulate abdominal fat (central obesity) which is demonstrated by a high waist:hip ratio (see Q4.4).

Central obesity is associated with unfavourable metabolic disturbances such as reduced insulin sensitivity, glucose intolerance and lipid abnormalities. This distribution of fat is generally considered a better predictor of both type 2 diabetes and cardiovascular risk than BMI. South Asians also have a prevalence of CHD around 50% higher than the national average, which cannot be explained by differences in smoking, blood pressure or cholesterol levels.

African-Caribbeans also have a high prevalence of type 2 diabetes. Although they are also prone to obesity, there is no evidence that they have any increased tendency towards a more central pattern of obesity than Europeans. Type 2 diabetes is, however, still associated with a higher waist:hip ratio in African-Caribbeans to the same extent as in Europeans (McKeigue et al., 1991). Typical blood lipid levels are more favourable in African-Caribbeans than in Europids and, as a consequence, mortality from CHD is lower, despite the high prevalence of diabetes. Several studies have, however, demonstrated that hypertension is more common and average blood pressure is higher in people of black African descent (Chaturvedi et al., 1993). They are therefore at greater risk of having a stroke.

Low-income Groups: Eating Healthily on a Tight Budget

Q3.103 What is the evidence that chronic disease is more prevalent in the poorer groups in our society?

Since the nineteenth century, life expectancy has increased dramatically in England and Wales, from 48 to 80 years in women and from 44 to 75 years in men. During the same time period, infant mortality has fallen from over 100 per 1000 to 6 per 1000 births. Improvements have not, however, been achieved at a similar rate among all social groups. The Black Report in 1980 (DHSS, 1980) showed ill-health and premature death from a wide range of diseases to be more prevalent among people with low income. The Acheson Report, produced by a Working Group chaired by Sir Donald Acheson in 1997, showed that these inequalities in health have persisted (Acheson, 1998).

Disorders such as obesity, diabetes, high blood pressure, and mortality from cardiovascular disease and cancers of the gastrointestinal tract, prostate, bladder and pancreas are all higher among the lower social classes, in both men and women. For example, death rates from CHD are around three times higher in unskilled men than among professionals even when conventional risk factors (e.g. smoking, cholesterol levels, alcohol consumption, physical activity) are taken into account (Department of Health, 2000b), and the gap has widened sharply in the last 20 years. At the same time, the number of people living in households that have 'relative poverty' has increased over the last 15 years. Between 13 and 14 million people currently live in households with an income below 50% of the UK average (<£120 per week). The recent Government White Paper, *Saving Lives: Our Healthier Nation* (Department of Health, 1999), recognised the increased risk of chronic diseases among the less well-off and outlined the social, economic and environmental determinants of these health inequalities. Many of the chronic diseases have a dietary component in their causation and considerable evidence supports the role of an unhealthy diet in the relationship between socioeconomic status and health.

Income has an important influence on both the type and the quality of food purchased. Diets of low-income households are characterised by less dietary variety compared with those of others in the population. The National Food Survey and other smaller surveys have reported substantial differences in the diets of the rich and the poor. Lower-income groups generally eat less of foods such as wholemeal bread, reduced-fat milk, poultry, carcass meat, fish, and fresh fruit and vegetables, and consume a higher proportion of white bread, whole milk, sugar, eggs, meat products and margarine. Although no single food can be regarded as 'healthy' or 'unhealthy', this pattern of consumption is less likely to conform to current dietary advice. In 1998, low-income households purchased less fruit, fewer fresh vegetables (other than potatoes) and fewer alcoholic drinks for home consumption, whereas they bought more whole milk and sugar (MAFF, 1999). Studies attempting to explain the different dietary patterns of different income groups have shown that knowledge about health and nutrition does not differ substantially. The major influences appear to be limited resources (money and cooking facilities), restricted access to shops and lack of confidence in preparing food (Shepherd et al., 1996).

Low-income groups have to spend a greater percentage of their total income on food (43% of the average income in low-income households versus 17% in high-income groups) (Shepherd et al., 1996). However, studies have shown that low-income families buy food more efficiently – they get more in terms of quantity and nutritional value for the money that they spend (Department of Health, 1996b). Shopping basket surveys have shown that foods such as fresh fruit and vegetables are a more expensive source of calories than cheaper, more filling alternatives such as biscuits, cakes and fattier cuts of meat. Moreover, the price of fruit and vegetables has increased more than the average over the last 20 years. A number of studies indicate that the cost of a diet that takes into account social factors, and is in line with current dietary advice, is substantially higher than the amount of money that people on low incomes have to spend (Hanes and De Looy, 1987). The diet recommended by the Department of Health may, therefore, be out of the reach of the poorest families. Young householders, unemployed people, those on benefit payments or very low incomes, and elderly people often have the greatest difficulties, the worst diets and, indeed, the poorest health expectations.

People in lower-income groups tend to pay more for their food because of the physical inaccessibility of large retail outlets such as out-of-town supermarkets. Many live in deprived neighbourhoods where comparatively few own cars and shopping facilities are poor. This necessitates expenditure on transport or payment of higher prices in small local shops. These 'food deserts' can increase a sense of social exclusion and widen health inequality. Shopping at small independent corner-shops can be as much as 60% more expensive than at supermarkets. Other issues such as poor facilities for cooking and a lack of cooking skills can exacerbate the problems.

A poor quality diet can affect health at all stages of the life course (Acheson, 1998). Infants from low-income households are less likely to be breast-fed and have a higher prevalence of anaemia. Inappropriate weaning is more common. In young children, poverty is associated with higher intakes of saturated fatty acids and sugar, and lower intakes of dietary fibre and most minerals and vitamins, especially the antioxidant vitamins. They have slower growth, are more likely to be obese, have higher blood lipids and have more dental caries. School-children in low-income households have lower intakes of many vitamins and minerals, including iron and calcium (especially in girls), which is associated with lower bone mass and more anaemia. Poor eating habits established during childhood often persist into adult life. Low socioeconomic status is linked with obesity in women and several other chronic diseases of adult life. Pregnant women in low-income households have lower energy and nutrient intakes, lower weight gains in pregnancy and a higher prevalence of anaemia. Low socioeconomic status is one of the most significant factors associated with low birthweight, a measure of poor pregnancy outcome and increased risk of disease in adult life. The risk of neural tube defects and stillbirths is also higher (Department of Health, 1996b).

Q3.104 Which nutrients are of most concern?

Associated with the lack of dietary variety are poorer nutrient profiles. Intakes of many nutrients are consistently found to be lower among low-income groups, including fibre, calcium, iron, zinc, riboflavin, niacin, vitamin C and β-carotene. Lower nutrient intakes in low or manual social classes have been consistently reported by small surveys and in the National Diet and Nutrition Surveys of children aged 1.5–4.5 years, 4–18 year olds, adults and older people (Gregory et al., 1990, 1995, 2000; Finch et al., 1998). The 1999 National Food Survey (MAFF, 2000) found intakes of energy and most nutrients to be the least for the lowest income groups (judged by income of the head of household). Although there is no evidence to suggest that those on low incomes have specific nutritional deficiencies, current nutritional knowledge about the protective role of antioxidant nutrients and other dietary factors suggests that there is scope for health gain if more vegetables, fruit, high-fibre cereals and fish were more accessible to poorer people. In common with other income groups, those on low income generally need to reduce their intake of fat, sugar and salt in order to meet dietary targets. They are, however, likely to face greater obstacles in doing so.

Q3.105 What practical and realistic advice can be offered?

With very careful shopping and the use of relatively cheap foods, e.g. dried pulses combined with vegetables, potatoes in place of bought pies, it is possible for a healthy diet to cost no more, and sometimes less, than an unhealthy one. Advice that can be given to improve the nutritional quality of the diet while saving money includes:

- Add extra pulses and vegetables to stews and casseroles to make meat go further.
- Have larger portions of potatoes, rice or starchy vegetables with smaller portions of meat or meat products.

- Meat does not have to be expensive to be nutritious; lean mince has a similar iron content to steak.
- Use as little fat or oil in cooking as possible and replace the calories with extra bread (particularly wholemeal), rice, potatoes or pasta.
- Spread butter or margarine thinly on thicker slices of bread.
- Plain yoghurt or fromage frais can replace packet toppings and cream.
- Use skimmed or semi-skimmed milk instead of whole milk.
- Make stale bread into breadcrumbs which can be used for meat loaves, rissoles and stuffing.
- By using strong cheese, the same flavour can be achieved with a much smaller amount; grating cheese can make it go further in sandwiches or salads.
- Fruit and vegetables that are in season are cheaper; buying smaller quantities will avoid wastage caused by spoilage; bruised or damaged fruit and vegetables are often cheaper but will deteriorate quicker and the vitamin content is lower.
- Buy fewer sweets, cakes and biscuits.
- Frozen vegetables are a useful alternative to fresh if freezer space is available; they can often be richer in vitamins than poorly stored fresh vegetables.
- Convenience foods can be very expensive; avoid those with relatively little nutritional value such as instant meals in pots; any savings can be offset against the cost of wholegrain products and fruit and vegetables.
- Left-overs can be used in another meal if stored properly.

Q3.106   How can the stresses of shopping on a tight budget be reduced?

The problem of shopping on a tight budget is compounded by the fact that small quantities of food are often relatively more expensive, prices in local shops are usually higher than in supermarkets and transport facilities are often poor in deprived areas. Low-income households may not have the money available to buy in sufficient quantities to justify a trip to a larger, cheaper shop. These problems are not easily resolved, but the following includes some advice that can be given:

- Make a list of items that are needed and stick to this to prevent impulse purchases.

- Forward planning will prevent emergency buys which can be more expensive.
- Sharing shopping with friends can reduce the transport costs.
- Large bargain packets can be shared with friends or neighbours; setting up small buying cooperatives can save money.
- Own supermarket brands may often be cheaper.
- Some goods are reduced in price late in the day or at weekends.
- Meat from the butcher can be cut to requirement rather than pre-packaged; this may be cheaper.

Q3.107   Are there suggestions for people with limited storage or cooking facilities?

Storage and cooking facilities can be very limited in low-income households and advice must be adjusted accordingly to ensure that it is appropriate. Keeping fuel costs down is also important and possible methods to achieve this include:

- Eat more raw fruit and vegetables.
- Buy smaller quantities to avoid wastage resulting from spoilage.
- Cook vegetables rapidly in a small amount of water.
- Stir fry vegetables in a small amount of oil.
- Grill tender lean meat rather than stewing tough fatty meats.
- Cooking several dishes at the same time can reduce fuel costs.
- Toasters use much less fuel than a grill on a cooker.

Q3.108   What can be done at a local level to help families living on a low income?

A number of local authorities have set up community projects to tackle the problems associated with food poverty. Local projects have used a wide variety of approaches to try to improve the access of low-income families to an adequate variety of good quality food, to provide information on how to make food choices and to provide the skills and facilities to prepare food. Activities have included:

- Food cooperatives/mobile shops.
- Cookery and shopping skills courses.
- Development and provision of healthy recipe leaflets developed locally and using readily available and economical ingredients.

- Food and nutrition education courses.
- Information leaflets about nutritional issues such as sensible snacking and budgeting for a healthier diet.
- Community cafés and lunch clubs providing healthy food at low cost.
- Meal provision for those with special needs, e.g. people with AIDS.
- Food coupons.
- Transport to shops.

Schools can also help by making their facilities accessible to allow projects such as community cafés, cookery courses or food-tasting sessions to be provided at a low cost. Where appropriate, the introduction of school breakfast programmes can ensure that children from low-income families are provided with a nutritious meal to start the day (see Q3.62).

The pricing policies of the major supermarket operators make available a range of own-brand products of reasonable quality at low prices and help those on a limited budget to attain a healthy diet. Low-priced fresh fruit and vegetables are usually offered as part of the low-priced own-label ranges or the extra value promotions, which have been introduced over the last couple of years. Typically, these fruit and vegetables are of equal nutritional quality to those sold at higher prices, but are sold at a lower price because, for example, they may be irregularly shaped. Other supermarkets guarantee that basic fruit and vegetables are available in extra value packs.

Action at the local level is the most effective way to assist people on low incomes in the first instance. However, local projects suffer from lack of funds, isolation, reliance on volunteers and absence of evaluation. This will be aided by the establishment of databases and networks to promote the exchange of information between projects that seem to alleviate food problems related to low income. Details for Sustain and the Health Department Agency are provided in the Useful Addresses list, p. 201.

Nutrition and Older People

Q3.109 What are the main nutritional issues?

As the proportion of older people in the population is increasing (by 2030 one-third of the UK population will be aged over 60 years), it is important that people are encouraged to remain healthy for as long as possible. This involves ensuring that older people have an adequate supply of nourishing food, particularly when they are ill and vulnerable.

October 1998 saw the publication of the National Diet and Nutrition Survey concerning people aged 65 years and over (Finch et al., 1998). This is a unique survey, which provides data on the dietary intake and nutritional status of 1275 free-living participants and 412 living in institutions. Data are also available on a range of anthropometric and biochemical parameters. Furthermore, a related dental survey was conducted among all the participants with some natural teeth and about 50% of those with none of their own teeth (Steele et al., 1998).

The survey showed that older people were, generally, adequately nourished but that a proportion of those studied had suboptimal intakes of several nutrients, including vitamin D, potassium and magnesium. The key public health issues highlighted in the report related to dental health, the relationship between B vitamin status and cardiovascular disease, and bone health (see Q3.112).

Some of those living in residential care had a poorer nutritional status (vitamin C in particular), as did those lacking their own teeth (regardless of whether they lived in institutions or were free-living in the community). Nutritional trends were also evident in relation to social class differences. The Government's White Paper, *Saving Lives: Our Healthier Nation* (Department of Health, 1999), recognises that health inequalities exist and need to be tackled. Among free-living subjects in the survey of older people, there was evidence that intakes of a range of nutrients were lower in manual households than those in non-manual households. In some cases, e.g. magnesium and potassium, intakes were quite low in comparison with the reference nutrient intake (RNI), particularly among women.

For a summary of the public health nutrition issues arising from the survey, see Buttriss (1999).

> Q3.110 Do requirements change with age and what is the impact on dietary recommendations?

The COMA report on Dietary Reference Values (Department of Health, 1991) gives nutritional recommendations for older people; these should be used as the basis of nutritional guidelines for this age group (see Tables 1.1–1.3).

Recommendations for intakes of fat, fatty acids, carbohydrate and dietary fibre are the same as for younger adults. It is particularly important, however, to ensure optimal intakes of fibre that will be helpful in alleviating symptoms of conditions such as constipation and diverticulosis, which can be common in older people (see Q2.1).

Recommendations for protein intake are marginally higher in older adults; the recommendation for men is 53.3 g/day and for women it is 46.5 g/day, over the age of 50 years (see Q2.7).

Vitamin and mineral reference values are also similar. An exception is iron, for which the recommendation is lower in older women, after the cessation of menstruation. In younger adults, there is no reference nutrient intake for vitamin D; however, those aged 50 years and over are advised to consume 10 µg of vitamin D per day.

In the USA, a higher calcium intake is recommended for older women, but experts in the UK do not believe this to be necessary in relation to bone health. Nevertheless, it is recognised that women at high risk of osteoporosis may benefit from a higher calcium intake (Department of Health, 1991) (see Q3.98).

Q3.111   Are people living alone in the community worse off nutritionally than
              those being cared for in institutions?

The Diet and Nutrition Survey (Finch et al., 1998) showed that, with one or two exceptions, intakes of vitamins and minerals in the institutionalised participants were lower than those of free-living participants (although they were generally above the RNI). However, for several nutrients, namely calcium, riboflavin and vitamin A, those in institutions fared better. These three nutrients are provided by milk, and milk/milk product intake was higher in those in residential care than in the free-living subjects.

When it came to biochemical and haematological indices of status, however, the findings were less satisfactory. A proportion of the free-living participants had low indices for folate, vitamin C, vitamin D and iron (magnesium and potassium were not included, but may be expected also to have been low on the basis of the intake data). The situation was typically worse in those in institutions, who had lower vitamin E, β-carotene and retinol indices. Status seemed to worsen with age, and status was typically better in non-manual compared with manual groups, and in those with their own teeth.

Q3.112   What are the main concerns?

Dental health

Those with no or few natural teeth ate a more restricted range of foods (Steele et al., 1998) influenced by their perceived inability to chew. The survey of older people confirmed an association between oral function and nutrient intake, and indicated that subjects without their own teeth, or with few teeth, were less likely to choose foods that need chewing, i.e. apples, raw carrots, toast, nuts and oranges. There was a clear association between oral function and nutritional status. For example, nutritional status with respect to iron, vitamin C, vitamin E and retinol was lower in those without teeth or with few teeth. Vitamin C status was particularly low in those living in institutions and there was an association between frequency of sugar intake and dental decay in those with teeth.

Table 3.6 illustrates that, among free-living participants, the absence of natural teeth had a significant impact on the intake of a range of nutrients. For those in institutions, nutrient intakes were generally lower anyway, and whether or not participants had their own teeth was less relevant to their nutrient intake.

In free-living subjects, vitamin C status was lower in those without natural teeth. Among those in institutions, the levels were considerably lower; in those without their own teeth, the data suggest that nearly half the subjects had an intake below the level regarded as signifying biochemical depletion.

Table 3.6 Effect of absence of own teeth on daily nutrient intake

	Free-living		Living in institutions	
	With teeth	Without	With teeth	Without
Energy (MJ)	7.39	6.62	6.95	7.07
Calcium (mg)	834	722	808	872
Iron (mg)	10.97	9.39	8.92	8.36
Vitamin A (µg)	1284	1036	1037	1032
Thiamin (mg)	2.30	1.36	1.15	1.20
Riboflavin (mg)	2.61	1.57	1.57	1.64
Vitamin C (mg)	81	60	47	55
Vitamin E (mg)	13.6	8.0	6.0	7.0

Source: Steele et al. (1998).

From a public health perspective, there is a need to encourage good oral health from childhood onwards, paying particular attention to use of fluoride toothpaste, oral hygiene and the frequency of sugar consumption (particularly between meals). More information on diet and oral health can be found in a British Nutrition Foundation Task Force Report on this subject (British Nutrition Foundation, 1999b).

Folate and vitamins B_{12} and B_6

The metabolism of folate, vitamin B_{12} and vitamin B_6 in the body is interlinked. There is particular interest in the metabolism of these three vitamins in relation to cardiovascular disease. Suboptimal status of folate and vitamins B_{12} and B_6 is correlated with a high plasma homocysteine concentration, which is now recognised as a predictor of CHD risk (see Q4.2). Homocysteine levels in the blood increase with age, and levels are relatively high in the UK compared with other parts of Europe and North America. Levels are higher in Scotland and northern England than in the south, as are mortality rates for cardiovascular disease.

In the survey (Steele et al., 1998), folate and vitamin B_6 were poorly supplied by some diets and are also known to be less well retained in the tissues of older people. Vitamin B_{12} absorption is also progressively impaired with age. These data, coupled with awareness of the importance of folate status during the early weeks of pregnancy, suggest that there is a need for practical advice on dietary sources of these nutrients for all age groups. It has been suggested that consideration should be given to the merits of fortifying foods with folic acid. The Government's advisory committee, COMA, recently reviewed the scientific evidence linking folate status and disease risk (Department of Health, 2000d). Their report recommended the universal fortification of flour at 240 µg/day per 100 g of food products as consumed. At this level, it was estimated that 40% of neural tube defects could be prevented without producing any risk of unacceptably high levels in any sectors of the population. In the USA, statutory fortification of flour has recently been adopted. Currently, voluntary fortification of a range of foods, particularly some breads and breakfast cereals, is carried out in the UK (see Q1.12). However, the issue of fortification is not as simple as it might appear at first sight. For example, fortification of foods with folic acid could potentially mask vitamin B_{12} deficiency in elderly people, which manifests as pernicious anaemia. The Government conducted a consultation exercise on the issue of folic acid fortification during 2000, the results of which are awaited.

Bone health

Osteoporosis is a significant factor in over 90% of fractures in people aged over 65 years. Such fractures are the cause of significant mortality, morbidity and economic cost. Vitamin D is important in bone metabolism, because it is needed for the absorption of calcium (see Q2.5 and Q2.22). It can be provided by skin synthesis or by the diet. Vitamin D levels fall in winter as skin synthesis ceases and, as a result, calcium absorption falls. This causes a change in serum-free calcium, which in turn stimulates parathyroid hormone secretion; this mobilises calcium from bone. As a result, fracture risk is increased. For more information, see Q3.98.

> Q3.113 What practical advice can be offered to improve calcium and vitamin D status?

Randomised controlled trials have shown that, in vulnerable groups, e.g. elderly women, calcium and vitamin D supplementation together reduce fracture risk (Department of Health, 1998a). Calcium alone has a more modest effect and vitamin D alone appears to be ineffective. A question that has been addressed by a recent COMA Working Group (Department of Health, 1998a) is whether there is sufficient evidence to warrant supplementation with either nutrient as a public health measure. COMA concluded that the current practice of fortifying flour with calcium should continue. It endorsed the current dietary reference value for vitamin D (10 µg/day for older people) and recommended that public and health professionals should be better informed about the importance of achieving adequate vitamin D status, including the appropriate use of supplements for those at most risk (see Q2.22 and Q2.37).

> Q3.114 Many older people have few natural teeth. How can this be overcome to ensure that a healthy diet is achieved?

Many older people have no natural teeth and may have to depend on false teeth. Where this is the case, it is important that the teeth are comfortable and properly fitting, and allow the wearer to bite and chew foods adequately. Full dental check-ups should be given regularly to ensure optimal dental function. For those who have some remaining teeth, good oral hygiene should be promoted. This means brushing the teeth regularly with a fluoride toothpaste. Sugary foods should not be consumed too frequently throughout the day and should, ideally, be restricted to mealtimes.

> Q3.115 What are the factors to look for that might signal a potential health problem?

There are a number of health problems that are common in old age. A healthy diet can contribute to alleviating some of these problems, particularly the following:

Constipation

Constipation is a common problem in older people, affecting one in five in this age group. Most at risk are those who have a poor diet and who take little exercise. Adequate intake of fibre and fluids should be promoted, as well as some physical activity if possible. Sources of fibre include wholegrain cereals, wholemeal flour and bread, wholegrain rice, pulses, fruit and vegetables (see Q2.1). If there are chewing difficulties, vegetables can be puréed to produce soups and fruit puréed to produce drinks. The addition of pure bran to foods is not recommended because it can interfere with the absorption of several minerals. Regular meals and snacks can help to ensure a good nutritional intake. Laxatives should not be the treatment of choice.

Anaemia

Iron-deficiency anaemia is common in older people, particularly those in residential care, where 52% of men and 39% of women have been reported to have low haemoglobin levels (Finch et al., 1998). This may be a result of poorer absorption of iron, e.g. the consumption of tea was high among the group with low haemoglobin levels and the tannins in tea inhibit the absorption of non-haem iron. Furthermore, gastric disorders are more common in older people, which can also interfere with efficient iron absorption or result in blood (and thereby iron) loss. The best food sources of iron are those containing iron in the haem form. Non-haem sources of iron can also make a useful contribution to overall intake (see Q2.6).

Diabetes

Around 1.4 million people in the UK currently suffer from diabetes (Diabetes UK, 2000). Between 75% and 90% of cases have type 2, or non-insulin-dependent diabetes, and 10–25% have type 1, or insulin-dependent diabetes. Dietary treatment of diabetes no longer involves the restriction of carbohydrate foods. Diabetic diets today are based on healthy eating principles (see Q4.13 and Q4.14). This means following a diet that is low in fat and high in carbohydrate, particularly complex carbohydrate. Intake of concentrated sources of sugars, such as sugary foods or drinks, should be limited, however. The use of special diabetic products should not be necessary. Regular meals and snacks should be encouraged. Physical activity should be promoted where possible and, if a person is overweight, advice to lose weight may be appropriate (see Q3.82, Q3.96 and Q4.10).

Overweight

Overweight and obesity affect a significant proportion of older people. In the Diet and Nutritional Survey of people aged 65 years and older, it was found that among free-living participants 67% of men and 63% of women were either overweight or obese (Finch et al., 1998). The corresponding figures for those living in residential care were 46% and 47% for men and women, respectively.

Some overweight older people, particularly those who have reduced mobility or osteoarthritis, may wish to lose weight. It is important, if reducing energy intake, to ensure that the diet is still properly balanced and provides sufficient vitamins and minerals to meet requirements. Any weight loss should be slow and gradual, at a rate of about 1–2 lb/week (see Q4.8).

Underweight

Underweight poses a greater risk to the health of older people than being overweight. This is a problem that is more prevalent in those living in residential care, where in the survey of people aged 65 years and over 16% of men and 15% of women in institutions were underweight. The corresponding figures for those living in the community were 3% for men and 6% for women, respectively.

Being underweight in old age has been shown to correlate with shorter survival (see British Nutrition Foundation, 1999a). Predisposing factors to undernutrition have been identified as living alone, being housebound, not having regular cooked meals, being on supplementary benefits, being of a lower social class, suffering from depression, having low mental test scores, having poor dentition, having chronic bronchitis or emphysema, having had a gastrectomy, experiencing swallowing difficulties, smoking and having alcohol problems. These risk factors do not necessarily indicate the need for intervention, but should be viewed as potential danger signs. The Malnutrition Advisory Group has developed a useful screening tool based on information about recent weight loss and weight/height measurments (Malnutrition Advisory Group, 2000)

The Caroline Walker Trust guidelines (1995), *Eating Well for Older People*, recommend that to reduce risk of undernutrition, vulnerable older people living in the community should be given a nutritional assessment by a member of the primary healthcare team. Older people in residential care should have their food and fluid needs assessed in the first week after admission and regularly thereafter. Body weight should be recorded regularly (at least once a month) using accurate scales. Unintended weight loss (or gain) of 3 kg (7 lb) or more should be referred, for assessment, to a state-registered dietitian.

Coronary heart disease and stroke

Coronary heart disease and stroke are significant causes of death and ill-health. They cause almost 115 000 deaths each year in England. Strokes caused over 54 000 deaths in 1997, most of which were in people over the age of 75 years (Department of Health, 1999).

Any strategy that limits the prevalence of these conditions will improve life expectancy and quality of life in older people. General healthy eating advice (see Q1.5–1.9) applies equally to older people, e.g. consuming a low-fat, high-carbohydrate diet that is rich in fruit and vegetables. Consumption of oil-rich fish is also recommended, at least one portion a week (see Q4.2).

Only for very old or frail people is this advice sometimes inappropriate; these people should be encouraged to eat whatever they can.

Chapter 4
Nutrition and the
Prevention/Treatment
of Diseases

As mentioned throughout the text, nutrition is closely related to many areas of health, from before conception to old age. This chapter examines the relationships more closely, but does not profess to offer expert guidance about other aspects of the individual diseases. The reader is referred to other specific texts for more detail.

Q4.1 What are the main chronic diseases in which nutrition may play a part?

Nutrition can play an important role in the prevention and treatment of a number of diseases. Coronary heart disease (CHD), stroke and cancer have been identified in a recent Government White Paper, *Our Healthier Nation* (Department of Health, 1999), as diseases that can be influenced by diet and lifestyle. Factors that are important for reducing risk are outlined in the sections below.

Obesity is another condition that can be affected by diet and lifestyle and is associated with a number of diseases, notably CHD, some cancers, type 2 (non-insulin-dependent) diabetes and osteoarthritis (see Q4.6). The prevalence of obesity is increasing at a phenomenal rate in the UK; appropriate dietary and lifestyle changes are needed to tackle this problem and would, in turn, reduce the incidence of obesity-related diseases.

Osteoporosis is another condition on which nutrition can have an important impact. This condition is likely to become more prevalent as the proportion of elderly people in the population increases; latest estimates suggest that the annual cost to the National Health Service for osteoporosis is £942 million (Department of Health, 1998a). Good nutrition and regular weight-bearing exercise early in life can optimise bone health and reduce risk of osteoporosis in later years (see Q3.98 and Q4.15).

There has been some suggestion that the severity or incidence of other diseases, such as arthritis, colds and flu, may be influenced by nutritional intake. More research is needed in these areas before firm recommendations can be made (see Q4.17).

Vegetarians have been shown to be at reduced risk of disease. Those following a vegetarian diet tend, however, to be more health conscious; also the vegetarian diet tends to be higher in fruit, vegetables and dietary fibre. It is unlikely that the simple exclusion of meat, in itself, would be the explanation (see Q4.18–4.22).

Finally, food allergy and intolerance are important areas to consider. For those who have a food allergy or intolerance, it is necessary to ensure the exclusion of the offending food while optimising nutritional intake, particularly in young children. For further information, see Q4.23–4.40.

Coronary Heart Disease (CHD)

Q4.2 What are the nutritional factors associated with CHD risk, and what are the associated dietary implications?

Two processes, atherosclerosis and thrombosis, together cause CHD, which may result in angina, myocardial infarction (heart attack) or sudden death. Atherosclerosis is the narrowing of the blood vessels in the heart caused by the deposition of fatty material, which becomes hardened and develops into a plaque. Thrombosis is the lodging of a blood clot in the narrowed blood vessel. This cuts off the blood supply to the dependent portion of heart muscle and the heart muscle becomes damaged.

Coronary heart disease is the most common cause of death in the UK and is a major cause of premature death (i.e. before the age of 65 years). It is more common in men than in women.

The risk of CHD can be reduced by following an appropriate diet, by stopping smoking and by taking regular exercise. Diet can beneficially affect the lipid (fat) levels in the blood. In the blood, lipids are carried by carrier proteins in the form of lipoproteins. There are a number of these, of differing composition. VLDL (very-low-density lipoproteins) particles carry mostly triacylglycerol (triglyceride) plus a small amount of cholesterol. Blood levels of

VLDL are highest after a meal and reflect the fat composition of the meal. A slow rate of clearance of VLDL is associated with obesity (especially centrally deposited obesity) and type 2 diabetes.

It is often forgotten that cholesterol is an essential component of cells, e.g. it has a crucial structural function especially in brain cells. Most of the cholesterol is carried in LDL particles and HDL particles. LDL particles carry cholesterol from the liver to the peripheral tissues, whereas HDL particles do the opposite. Although dietary cholesterol intake has an effect on the amount of cholesterol circulating in the blood, most of the cholesterol is in fact synthesised within the body in response to factors such as the level of saturated fatty acid intake (see Q2.4). It is also governed to some extent by genetic factors, e.g. some individuals are predisposed to familial hypercholesterolaemia. A high level of LDL-cholesterol is a marker of increased risk of CHD, whereas a high level of HDL-cholesterol decreases the risk of CHD. The levels of these fractions in the blood depend partly on genetic factors, but are also influenced by diet and, in the case of HDL-cholesterol, physical activity levels and alcohol intake.

High intakes of fat, and in particular saturated fatty acids, increase blood levels of LDL-cholesterol. The main sources of saturates in the UK diet are fat spreads (e.g. butter, hard margarine, lard) and products made from them (e.g. pastry and baked goods), fatty meat and meat products, and dairy products made from whole milk. To reduce intake of saturated fatty acids, lean cuts of meat should be selected instead of fatty cuts, reduced fat spreads and dairy products should be chosen, and the intake of pastry and baked goods should be reduced. High intakes of dietary cholesterol can increase blood LDL-cholesterol; however, for most people dietary cholesterol intake is not a problem. High intakes of *trans*-fatty acids, found in hard margarine, processed foods, cakes and biscuits, can lower HDL-cholesterol levels in the blood to some extent.

Monounsaturated fatty acids (e.g. found in olive oil and rapeseed oil) and *n-6* polyunsaturated fatty acids (e.g. found in sunflower and corn oils) can help lower LDL-cholesterol levels, and so reduce the risk of CHD. Monounsaturated fatty acids also raise HDL-cholesterol levels. This is the major type of fat in the so-called Mediterranean diet, which is associated with a lower incidence of CHD. The long-chain *n-3* polyunsaturates found in oil-rich fish have little effect on blood cholesterol. For a more detailed description of the types of fatty acids in foods, see Q2.4.

Fruit and vegetables contain substances called antioxidants that can help prevent the oxidation of LDL-cholesterol (see Q2.8). It is this oxidation of LDL that is now thought to be a crucial factor in the development of atherosclerosis. A detailed explanation can be found in a British Nutrition Foundation Briefing Paper, *Coronary Heart Disease 2* (British Nutrition Foundation, 1992). Antioxidants include vitamin E, vitamin C, β-carotene, selenium, copper and manganese. Research has shown a direct link between high consumption of fruit and vegetables and lower risk of CHD (Department of Health, 1994b). A review of this research will be presented in a British Nutrition Foundation Task Force Report due to be published in 2001.

Another dietary component that may have a favourable effect on blood cholesterol levels is soluble fibre (see Q2.1).

Eating oil-rich fish, such as mackerel, salmon and herring, has been shown to reduce the risk of CHD (see British Nutrition Foundation, 1999c). Various mechanisms have been proposed but the most likely is that the very-long-chain *n*-3 fatty acids present in oil-rich fish reduce triacylglycerol levels in blood. They may also help prevent clot formation by influencing the types of prostaglandins formed (for more details, see British Nutrition Foundation, 1999c). At least one serving of oil-rich fish per week is recommended for the general population (Department of Health, 1994b) and those with heart disease may benefit from higher intakes.

High blood pressure is a risk factor for CHD. Blood pressure may be raised in people who are obese, have a high salt intake, drink too much alcohol (more than 2–3 units/day for women and 3–4 units/day for men), take little or no exercise, or smoke cigarettes.

Recently, interest has developed in other substances that may have a protective effect against CHD. These phytochemicals (or plant chemicals), found in foods such as fruit, vegetables, tea, red wine and soya, are thought to have an important antioxidant effect and may also act by other mechanisms (see Q2.9). Therefore, although they are not currently considered to be 'nutrients', they may be important for optimal health. This area merits further research and is the subject of a British Nutrition Foundation Task Force, due to report in 2001.

To reduce risk of CHD, the dietary advice for most people in the UK is summarised in Box 4.1.

Box 4.1 Summary of dietary advice to reduce risk of CHD

To reduce consumption of all types of fat, e.g. by selecting lean cuts of meat and lower-fat dairy products, by reducing use of oil and full-fat spreads (margarine, butter), by eating fewer fried foods, and by moderating consumption of high fat foods such as cakes, biscuits, crisps and savoury snacks

To opt for oils/spreads that are higher in monounsaturated fatty acids and lower in saturated fatty acids

To include more fruit and vegetables in the diet – aim to have at least five portions of a variety of fruits and vegetables each day

To include oil-rich fish in the diet once per week (those with heart disease may benefit from higher intakes)

To include more starchy foods in the diet, e.g. bread, potatoes, rice and pasta, so that at least 50% of energy intake comes from carbohydrate

To drink alcohol sensibly, i.e. no more than two to three drinks per day for women and no more than three to four drinks per day for men

---

Cancer

Q4.3 Is there a link between diet and cancer?

Cancer, along with coronary heart disease, is one of the main causes of death in the UK. A recent report, which looked at dietary and nutritional factors in the development of cancer (Department of Health, 1998c), recognised that certain dietary characteristics can influence the development of cancer at certain sites. A number of key recommendations were made to reduce risk of the development of cancer. These are:

Maintain a healthy body weight

Obesity has been associated with increased risk of cancer, particularly breast cancer in postmenopausal women. There is also an increased risk of endometrial, uterine, ovarian and gallbladder cancers in obese women and increased risk of colon, rectal and prostate cancers in obese men (see Q3.88).

Increase intakes of a wide variety of fruit and vegetables

A higher intake of fruit and vegetables is associated with reduced risk of cancer at certain sites, particularly the colon, rectum and stomach. Everyone should aim to increase their intakes of fruit and vegetables to at least five portions a day to protect against the development of some cancers (see Department of Health, 2000c, for policy recommendations). At this stage it is not known precisely which components are most important. For this reason, incorporation of a variety of types into the diet is especially important. This situation also means that advice should focus on foods rather than supplements (see below).

Intake of red and processed meat should not increase

There is some evidence of a link between consumption of red and processed meat and colorectal cancer (Department of Health, 1998c). A reduction in meat consumption may, however, have adverse nutritional implications – in particular, iron intake may be reduced. For this reason, it is recommended that the current average intake of red and processed meat (about 90 g/day cooked weight, or 8–10 portions a week) should not rise.

Increase intake of non-starch polysaccharides (fibre) from a variety of sources

There is moderately consistent evidence that a higher intake of dietary fibre has the potential to lower the risk of colorectal and pancreatic cancer. Intakes among adults should be increased from the current average of 12 g/day to the recommended 18 g/day (see Q2.1). There is no specific recommendation for children, but younger children need proportionally less.

All the above recommendations should be followed in the context of a balanced diet (see Q1.6). Additional advice was given by the COMA working group to avoid intake of β-carotene supplements as a means of protecting against cancer and to exercise caution in the use of high-dose purified supplements of other micronutrients (see Q2.11) (Department of Health, 1998c). The advice regarding β-carotene was a result of the unexpected finding in several intervention studies that supplements increased the risk of lung cancer in male smokers.

Obesity

Q4.4 How is obesity defined?

The definition of obesity is based on risk to health. Body mass index

(BMI) is a commonly used measure to assess whether an individual is clinically obese. This is calculated using:

BMI = Weight (kg)/[Height (m) × Height (m)]

Although the BMI ranges are applicable to adult men and women, they are not satisfactory for children, adolescents or elderly people, in whom the proportion of lean body mass is changing. This index is best applied to the age range 19–65 years and a BMI between 20 and 25 is considered desirable in this age range. A BMI in adults of 25–30 indicates that an individual is overweight; a BMI of above 30 indicates that an individual is clinically obese and, as such, the condition constitutes a risk to health. The Child Growth Foundation has published some suggested BMI ranges for children.

A simpler way of determining health risk in adults is to measure waist circumference. A waist measurement of over 94 cm (37 inches) in men and 80 cm (32 inches) in women is associated with increased risk to health. A waist measurement of over 102 cm (40 inches) in men and 88 cm (35 inches) in women is associated with a substantial risk to health.

Q4.5 How common is obesity in the UK today?

Between 1980 and 1997, the prevalence of obesity increased in England from 6% to 17% in men and from 8% to 20% in women. The number of men and women who are now overweight/obese is 62% and 53% respectively (figures published for 1997) (British Nutrition Foundation, 1999a). Obesity is a reversible condition; action is needed now to prevent and treat this problem.

The pattern throughout the UK is fairly similar, with little regional variation. In general, BMI increases with age in both men and women up to the age of 64 years, then decreases slightly in older age groups. The relationship between BMI and social class varies with sex. In women, BMI tends to be higher in the manual social classes than in the non-manual social classes. In men, the pattern is less clear (Figure 4.1). Furthermore, an inverse association has been reported between educational attainment and BMI, particularly among women (Department of Health, 1994a). Vegetarians have a lower BMI than omnivores, although this is likely to result from factors other than the exclusion of meat from the diet (see Q4.22).

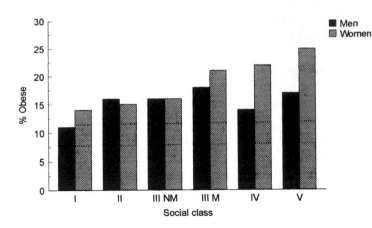

Figure 4.1 The relationship between obesity and social class. NM, non-manual; M, manual. (Source: Prescott-Clarke and Primatesta, 1998.)

A recent report published by the British Nutrition Foundation (1999a) details the factors responsible for the development of obesity and proposes suitable methods of prevention and treatment, on both a population and an individual level.

Q4.6 Are there health risks associated with being clinically obese?

The fact that obesity is a serious medical condition is being increasingly recognised. Obese people are at increased risk of heart disease, hypertension, type 2 (non-insulin-dependent) diabetes, gallstones, osteoarthritis of weight-bearing joints, sleep apnoea, reproductive disorders and some cancers. It is important that obesity is given more prominence as a risk factor for disease.

Q4.7 Is obesity a result of a slow metabolism?

The 'old myth' that obesity occurs as a result of a low metabolic rate is unfounded. One of the few statements about obesity that can be made with absolute certainty is that obesity can occur only when energy intake remains higher than energy expenditure for an extended period of time. In other words, where there is a chronic displacement of the energy balance equation ('energy in' minus 'energy out' = change in body energy stores).

Environmental changes that have occurred over the last few years, such as a more sedentary lifestyle and the ready availability of energy-dense foods, are the most likely underlying factors in the increasing prevalence of obesity. There are studies that have shown small differences in metabolism between obese subjects and their lean counterparts, but these differences are very subtle and are far outweighed by the impact of environmental influences and behavioural factors (British Nutrition Foundation, 1999a). A key strategy in tackling the rising prevalence of obesity must be education about the need for positive lifestyle changes. Health professionals should provide advice both for individuals and at a population level.

Q4.8 What is the role of diet in the prevention and treatment of obesity?

Predisposition to obesity has often been associated with intakes of high-fat foods. There does seem to be an increased liking for high-fat foods in those predisposed to obesity, e.g. obese people, formerly obese people, non-obese people with a high BMI, children of obese parents and restrained eaters.

There are a wide variety of dietary interventions available for the treatment of obesity, including low-calorie diets, very-low-calorie diets, milk diets and novel diets. Unfortunately, with many diets, long-term follow-up shows that much of the weight lost is regained. For dietetic success, it is important to focus on the patient's individual needs, to set realistic goals, to instigate small achievable changes rather than large changes, and to focus on weight maintenance (once the desired amount of weight has been lost). Dietary strategies form an important part of the treatment of obesity. See hda-online.org.uk for information on successful interventions.

Q4.9 Is behavioural therapy important?

A deeper understanding of weight control and problem-solving among health professionals should be encouraged. In terms of behavioural therapy, flexible long-term strategies that deal with both diet and activity should be promoted. Emotional issues also need to be addressed. 'Body image dissatisfaction', for example, is highly correlated with obesity, particularly among women and younger people; ethnicity can also influence body image. Cognitive behavioural treatments are increasingly addressing the reduction of 'body image distress'; this can make a significant contribution to well-being. See hda-online.org.uk.

Q4.10 Is physical activity important?

In terms of prevention, the development of new strategies to promote an environment that is 'user-friendly' in terms of activity is important. This will require action from the Government, local authorities and health authorities to provide affordable recreational facilities and safe environments for walking, jogging or cycling.

There are many benefits of exercise, which go far beyond weight control, e.g. exercise can reduce depression, anxiety and stress, enhance mood and self-esteem, and improve sleep quality. There is an increasing trend in inactivity in the UK at the present time, especially in children, and this is a problem that needs to be tackled. Recommendations for obese people, in terms of activity, are: that the amount of time spent in sedentary activities should be reduced; vigorous activity should be avoided, bouts of longer periods of moderate and sustained exercise are more beneficial; and more weight-bearing movement should be encouraged.

Q4.11 What about using drugs to treat obesity?

Where methods such as dietary intervention, behavioural therapy and promotion of physical activity have failed to achieve a weight loss of 10% after 3 months of managed care, it may be appropriate to consider an anti-obesity drug. For example, Orlistat, which is a pancreatic lipase inhibitor, has been available in the UK since 1998. Sibutramine, which promotes satiety, is currently licensed for use in Germany but is not available in the UK. The recent withdrawal of fenfluramine and dexfenfluramine, as a result of safety concerns, underlies the importance of continued monitoring of anti-obesity drugs to ensure that there are no adverse effects.

Q4.12 What are the key policy recommendations to prevent and treat obesity in the future?

Changes need to be promoted both in people and in the environment in which they live. There are four key issues that need to be addressed. These are:

1. Obesity is now a serious health problem in an increasing proportion of the population; action is now needed to prevent a further increase in prevalence.

2. Part of the solution involves changing the national diet to include more foods of a low-energy density such as fruit and vegetables.
3. Another part of the solution is to change the national lifestyle to include more physical activity, particularly opportunistic exercise such as using the stairs, and walking rather than using the car or bus for short distances. Strategies should address the needs of all segments of the population, but especially children.
4. Strategies are now needed for both prevention and treatment of obesity; one strategy can not be expected to be effective for both objectives.

Four key groups were identified in the British Nutrition Foundation's (1999a) Task Force report on obesity, which made key recommendations to tackle this problem. These groups are policy-makers, those who can prevent obesity, those who can treat obesity, and communicators and educators.

Policy-makers, such as the Government, local authorities and health authorities, are in the best position to alter the environmental factors that have led to the increase in obesity. For example, people who promote miracle weight-loss cures often undermine the work of responsible healthcare professionals, such as dietitians, doctors and nurses. New legislation to help control false weight-loss claims would be useful. It may also be helpful if local health authorities provided endorsement for those commercial slimming clubs in their area that provide a good service. A change in national patterns of physical activity also needs to be promoted by policy-makers. It is important to ensure that affordable recreational facilities and safe environments for walking, jogging or cycling are available for the whole population. In particular, children should be encouraged to view physical activity as a normal part of their everyday life.

Those in a position to help prevent obesity include public health directors, GPs, dietitians, practice nurses and other healthcare professionals, schools, teachers, parents and carers, slimming clubs, and the diet, food and fitness industries. Health professionals can play a role in educating the public about the range of weight-for-height at which health risks become significant, i.e. a BMI of over 30. The food and catering industry should continue to promote foods of a low-energy density and ensure that these are readily available. Finally, school authorities should ensure that there are opportunities for physical activity for children, in order to establish good habits from an early age.

Those who treat obesity include many of those involved in prevention, in particular healthcare professionals and the diet and slimming industry. Healthcare professionals, who have one-to-one contact, are especially well placed to give advice to overweight and obese people and to stress the benefits that weight loss will bring. It should be pointed out, however, that it is worse to treat obesity inadequately than not to treat it at all. Those involved in the treatment of obesity need to ensure that they have the required skills, otherwise patients should be referred to the most appropriate person. The essential steps in managing weight loss are as follows:

- to clarify the costs and benefits to the obese individual of weight loss;
- to choose the treatment most likely to achieve the desired result;
- to ensure that a competent and sympathetic health-care professional is available to review progress (normally every 1–4 weeks);
- to refrain from making exaggerated claims about the rapidity or efficacy of weight-loss programmes;
- to provide an indefinite after-weight-loss service to ensure weight maintenance.

Communicators include journalists and health educators. The Task Force urged journalists to ensure that they check the validity of press releases and other sources of information before publishing their stories. It can be all too easy simply to extract copy from a press release that extols the virtues of a particular weight-loss 'cure' without properly checking the facts. It is important that stories reported in the press, on the radio and on TV do not mislead and confuse the public (see Q5.1).

Diabetes

Q4.13 What is diabetes?

Diabetes is an endocrine disorder that results in partial or complete lack of the hormone insulin. Insulin is the hormone that controls blood glucose levels. Symptoms associated with diabetes include polydipsia (excessive thirst), polyuria (excessive urine production) and rapid weight loss. A blood glucose measurement of over 11.1 mmol/l is diagnostic of the condition. Diabetes can be divided into the following categories:

1. Primary diabetes mellitus:
   - type 1 (insulin dependent)
   - type 2 (non-insulin dependent)
   - obese
   - non-obese
   - gestational.
2. Secondary diabetes mellitus, resulting from:
   - pancreatic disease
   - endocrine diseases such as Cushing's syndrome
   - metabolic disorders
   - drug usage.
3. Impaired glucose tolerance.

Types 1 and 2 diabetes account for the majority of cases. Type 2 diabetes is often associated with obesity, especially where the fat is distributed centrally.

Q4.14 How is diabetes treated?

Type 1 diabetes is treated with a combination of insulin injections and diet. Type 2 diabetes is treated either with oral hypoglycaemic drugs and diet or by diet alone. The main aims of dietetic treatment are:

- to maintain blood glucose levels within as normal a range as possible;
- to minimise the risk of hypoglycaemia;
- to achieve weight loss in overweight and obese people;
- to prevent complications in the long term; these include heart disease (see Q4.2), nephropathy (damage to the kidney), neuropathy (damage to the nerves) and retinopathy (damage to the eye).

Dietary advice for people with diabetes is these days based on healthy eating guidelines (see Q1.5–1.10). The key points are as follows:

- Eat regular meals and snacks.
- Eat the right balance of foods, in line with the 'Balance of Good Health' (see Figure 1.2).
- Maintain a body weight within the ideal range; for overweight and obese people with diabetes, weight loss should be an important part of treatment (see Q4.8–4.12).
- Avoid excessive intakes of foods that are high in fat.
- Avoid an excessive intake of sugary foods and drinks.
- Complete avoidance of sugar is no longer necessary in a person with well-controlled diabetes, but intake of sugary foods and drinks should be limited.
- Special diabetic foods are not necessary – they can be high in calories and are often expensive, and as such they should not be encouraged.
- Avoid drinking on an empty stomach, or drinking excessively, because alcohol can cause blood sugar levels to fall too low.
- Regular exercise is important, particularly if trying to lose weight.

For further information, contact Diabetes UK (see Useful addresses). The reader is also referred to *Diabetes: A Handbook for Community Nurses*, by Zoe Crosby and Eileen Turner (another title in this series).

Osteoporosis

Q4.15   What are the nutritional factors associated with an increased risk of osteoporosis?

Osteoporosis is a disease characterised by loss of bone mass and increased risk of bone fracture. Osteoporosis can be classified as follows:

- Juvenile: this can occur in children aged 8–15 years; it is very rare.
- Young adult: this is sometimes seen in pregnancy but, again, is very rare.
- Postmenopausal (type I): occurs in women after the menopause, up to the eighth decade of life.
- Senile (type II): occurs in men and women over 75 years of age.
- Secondary: occurs as a secondary condition, e.g. in anorexia nervosa or after chronic steroid usage.

A recent report by COMA on Nutrition and Bone Health (Department of Health, 1998a) identified the following nutritional factors as being important:

- A healthy lifestyle to maintain bone health should be encouraged at all ages. A varied diet combined with regular weight-bearing physical activity is the best way forward.
- No change is recommended in the current dietary reference value for calcium (see Table 1.3).
- Dietary means of achieving an adequate calcium intake should be encouraged.
- The current practice of fortifying white flour with calcium should continue.
- Current dietary reference values for vitamin D are endorsed (see Table 1.2).

The public and health professionals should be better informed about the importance of achieving adequate vitamin D status. Particular consideration should be given to:

- infants, young children and pregnant women from Asian families;
- older people who are housebound;
- people who rarely go out of doors, or who wear clothes to conceal their bodies fully when they do go out.

For further information, see Q3.98, Q3.101 and Q5.12. The reader is also referred to *Rheumatology: A Handbook for Community Nurses* by Sarah Ryan and Jackie Hill (another title in this series).

Arthritis

Q4.16 Can diet alleviate the symptoms of arthritis?

Rheumatoid arthritis is the most common type of arthritis; it occurs more often in women and is usually associated with middle age, although, rarely, it can affect children. It has been reported that very-long-chain n-3 fatty acids can moderately decrease pain and morning stiffness in people with rheumatoid arthritis. These fatty acids are found in oil-rich fish (see Q2.4 and Q4.2) and in fish-oil supplements. Although supplements have been shown to alleviate symptoms to some extent in some individuals, more research is needed to evaluate the potential role of oil-rich fish in the diets of people with the condition. This subject has been reviewed in a recent British Nutrition Foundation Briefing Paper (1999c).

Osteoarthritis of weight-bearing joints is often associated with obesity, particularly in middle-aged women. The risk of osteoarthritis is related to the total amount of body fat, rather than fat distribution. Weight loss can alleviate symptoms (see Q4.8–4.12). (See also Ryan and Hill – as above.)

Colds and Flu

Q4.17 Can diet influence the chances of catching a cold or flu?

There has been much debate in recent years about the role of diet in preventing and curing the common cold and flu. Particular focus has been placed on vitamin C, and this vitamin is now added to numerous remedies for colds and flu (see Q2.20), and a large number of scientific studies have investigated its effect. Overall, it can be concluded that supplements will not prevent these viruses exerting their effects, but an increase in intake of vitamin C may help alleviate the severity of the symptoms, particularly if previous intake of vitamin C had been inadequate. Vitamin C-containing foods include citrus and soft fruit, green vegetables and potatoes (especially new potatoes). Megadosing on several grams per day, by taking high-dose supplements, has not been shown to prevent colds. It may occasionally lead to diarrhoea, increased production of oxalate (predisposing those with a high propensity for oxalate synthesis to kidney stones) and 'systematic conditioning', where sudden cessation of high intakes could lead to subsequent (temporary) deficiency through enhanced turnover established during the period of high intake. Studies have shown that tissues are saturated at intakes of about 200 mg/day (the RNI for adults is 40 mg/day).

Vegetarianism

Q4.18 How common is vegetarianism and what are the different types of diet adopted?

The term 'vegetarianism' encompasses a wide range of eating patterns. Table 4.1 lists the main categories of vegetarian diets.

Table 4.1 Categories of vegetarian diets

Diet	Description
Semi or partial vegetarian	This is not a strictly vegetarian diet, but involves the partial avoidance of animal foods. Red meat may be avoided but fish and perhaps poultry are often still eaten
Lacto-ovo vegetarian	Dairy products and eggs are consumed but fish, meat, poultry and their products are avoided. Ingredients derived from these sources are also usually avoided, e.g. gelatine and rennet
Lacto-vegetarian	As for lacto-ovovegetarian, but also exclude eggs from the diet
Vegan	Exclude all animal-derived products and ingredients
Macrobiotic	Similar to a vegan diet in many ways, with the bulk of the nutritional intake derived from cereals, vegetables and pulses. There is a limited intake of fruits, nuts and seeds; a small amount of fish may be eaten occasionally. There are various levels of food exclusion, at the most extreme level only brown rice is eaten

It has been estimated that 2–3% of the UK population are vegetarians, although within some age groups it is becoming an increasingly popular way of eating (see British Nutrition Foundation, 1995), e.g. among teenage girls, as many as 13% have been reported to be following a vegetarian eating pattern.

There have been concerns expressed about the nutritional adequacy of a vegetarian diet, especially for young children. However, with careful planning, a good nutritional intake can be achieved. It is particularly important that people turning to a vegetarian eating pattern for the first time get sound information about how to plan such a diet, so that the nutrients that would normally be available via meat (e.g. protein, iron, zinc and vitamin B_{12}) are provided by other foods, e.g. sources of iron suitable for vegetarians include pulses, green vegetables and bread made from iron-fortified flour. The more restrictive the diet, the more chance there is of a nutritional deficiency, so vegan diets in particular should be planned with care. The extreme restriction of food intake seen with some types of macrobiotic diet (e.g. consumption of only brown rice at the most extreme level) should be avoided, because nutritional deficiencies will almost certainly occur.

Q4.19   What are the guidelines for formulating a nutritionally balanced
vegetarian diet?

A well-balanced vegetarian diet, which includes a wide variety of
foods, will provide all the nutrients needed for health. Simply excluding meat from the diet, however, without replacing the nutrients that
meat would have provided, may result in low intakes of some essential nutrients.

The principles outlined in Q1.5–1.9 should be followed with any
style of eating and the 'Balance of Good Health' (see Figure 1.2) is a
useful guide to follow.

Q4.20   Are there any nutritional risks associated with this style of eating?

Although vegetarian diets may provide adequate amounts of iron,
there is a risk of poor iron status because the non-haem iron in plant
foods is less well absorbed than the haem iron in meat. Substances
such as phytates and oxalates may further inhibit absorption.
Sources of iron suitable for vegetarians include fortified cereals,
pulses, nuts and dark-green vegetables. If these foods are eaten
alongside foods that contain good amounts of vitamin C, such as
citrus fruit (and juice) and soft fruit, absorption of the non-haem iron
will be enhanced (see Q2.6).

Serum vitamin B_{12} concentrations have also been found to be
low in some vegetarians, particularly those who avoid all animal
products. Vitamin B_{12} is found naturally only in foods of animal
origin, so vegans must ensure that fortified foods, e.g. breakfast
cereals with added vitamin B_{12} or B_{12}-fortified vegetable extract,
are included in their diets; otherwise, they should take a supplement (see Q2.16).

Vegetarian, and in particular vegan, diets also have the potential
to be low in zinc, because the best sources of this mineral are meat,
poultry, seafood and milk (see Q2.29). In addition, bioavailability of
zinc can be reduced by phytate, oxalate and soy products, although it
is possible that vegetarians may adapt to a high-fibre high-phytate
diet by increasing the proportion of dietary zinc absorbed as it passes
through the small intestine. Lacto-ovovegetarians will obtain zinc
from consumption of milk and dairy products. For those following a
vegan diet, foods such as cereals, pulses and nuts should be included
regularly to ensure adequate zinc intake.

Those who avoid dairy products may have lower intakes of calcium, because milk and milk products are a major source of this mineral in the UK diet (together providing more than half of the calcium consumed in the average diet). Particular care is needed with the diets of vegan children and vegan lactating mothers. Sources of calcium suitable for vegans include breads and cereal foods (made from fortified flour), some green vegetables, e.g. broccoli (but not spinach – the calcium is not bioavailable), and some nuts and seeds, e.g. sesame seeds and peanuts (see Q2.5).

Q4.21 Are vegetarian and vegan diets suitable for young children?

It is possible to bring children up on a vegetarian or vegan diet that is nutritionally adequate. However, it should be remembered that young children require a nutrient-dense diet and can be at risk of poor nutritional intakes if the diet is not planned carefully. Deficiency of iron, vitamin D and vitamin B_{12}, and a low energy intake have been reported in vegetarian children in some studies. The more restrictive the diet, the more likely nutritional deficiencies become (see Q3.45). For those parents wishing to bring up young children on a vegan diet, advice from a qualified dietitian should be sought.

Q4.22 Are vegetarians generally healthier than meat eaters?

It is widely reported that vegetarians are healthier than meat eaters. Certainly, there is some evidence of lower morbidity and mortality rates in vegetarians. It is not clear, however, from the current scientific evidence, if it is simply the exclusion of meat from the diet that is protective or whether, as is more likely, a number of other dietary and lifestyle factors are involved. Vegetarians tend to be more health conscious than meat eaters, e.g. they often smoke less and exercise more. In addition, a vegetarian diet typically contains more fruit, vegetables and dietary fibre, factors that may help to protect against cancer and CHD.

Allergy and Intolerance

Q4.23 How are adverse reactions to food categorised?

'Adverse reactions to food' can be used as an umbrella term to cover food aversion, food intolerance and food poisoning (Figure 4.2).

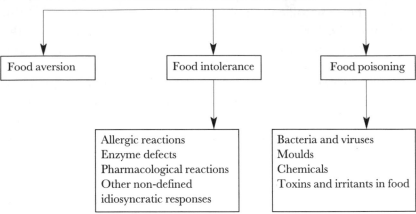

Figure 4.2 Categories of adverse reactions to food.

'Food intolerance' is the term used to describe a range of responses to food, including allergic reactions. This umbrella term also includes adverse reactions resulting from enzyme deficiencies such as lactose intolerance, and pharmacological reactions to food components such as vasoamines or caffeine. From time to time, cases of food intolerance occur that cannot be attributed to any of these categories and these are categorised as non-defined idiosyncratic responses, e.g. some foods contain naturally occurring toxins or substances that can irritate the lining of the intestine of some individuals. Dislike and subsequent avoidance of foods are referred to as food aversion. Although symptoms may be similar to those associated with true food intolerances, such reactions are psychosomatic and do not occur when the food or food ingredient is administered in a disguised form. The term 'food poisoning' is used to describe a disturbance of the gastrointestinal tract after the consumption of contaminated food or water.

True food allergy most often affects young children, but the majority outgrow this before they go to school. It is important to recognise that, in babies and young children in particular, development of specific antibodies to environmental allergens, especially those encountered in early life, is a normal physiological response via which tolerance to the environment is developed.

Q4.24 What is food allergy and why does it occur?

The term 'allergy' is often used inappropriately. An allergy is a specific form of intolerance involving the abnormal reaction of a person's immune system to a substance, e.g. a pollen grain or food constituent, which would have no harmful effect in most people. The immune system protects the body from harmful foreign proteins, antigens, by generating a response to eliminate them or develop tolerance towards them. An immune response can involve various cell types and a variety of proteins that can trigger inflammatory reactions. These can be used in eliminating the protein. On the other hand, an antibody may be produced against an antigen. An antibody is a protein (an immunoglobulin) that specifically binds with the antigen to deactivate it. Excessive or abnormal responses are associated with allergy. A person can display an allergic reaction to a substance only after previously being sensitised to it through initial exposure. The location within the body of signs and symptoms of food allergy is variable, and to some extent reflects the route of exposure. Signs and symptoms also vary in their timing and severity.

Genetic predisposition and a susceptible immune system, notably elevated blood levels of immunoglobulin E (IgE), are the most important determinants of allergic disease. Exposure to environmental factors, including dietary components, is secondary to these. Children with high blood IgE levels often suffer from asthma and hayfever and may also be allergic to one or more of the following: cows' milk, soya, eggs, citrus fruit or fish.

Different forms of allergic reactions can be classified according to the mechanism of the reaction. IgE-mediated (fast) reactions are immediate, can be severe and are mediated by specific antibodies – IgE – interacting with mast cells. The mast cells are present below the surface of the skin and in the membranes lining the nose, respiratory tract, eyes and intestine. A substance known as histamine and other inflammatory substances present in mast cells are then released and cause symptoms such as a runny nose, asthma, dilatation of blood vessels and flushing, swelling (e.g. of the lips) or difficulty in breathing. The severity of these reactions can vary, but severe responses are known as anaphylactic shock, which can result in unconsiousness and death. Peanuts are well known for causing this type of extreme reaction. Other foods that are known very occasionally to cause a severe IgE-mediated reaction are nuts, seeds (e.g. sesame), eggs, milk and shellfish.

Non-IgE-mediated (delayed) allergic reactions are mediated by the cells of the immune system or are mediated by immune complexes (antigen/antibody complexes), which continue to circulate in the bloodstream or are deposited in tissue. The best defined example of this type of reaction is coeliac disease. More detail can be found in a British Nutrition Foundation Briefing Paper on this subject (British Nutrition Foundation, 2000). Adverse reactions to food are also the subject of a British Nutrition Foundation Task Force, which is due to complete its deliberations in 2001.

Q4.25 Is it true that allergy is becoming more common?

There is consistent evidence that allergic reactions to non-food inhalant allergens, e.g. hayfever and asthma, are on the increase. It is speculated that food allergy may also be more common; however, there is no evidence to support this assumption. The prevalence of food allergy in the UK at present is estimated to be 1.4% of the population (see British Nutrition Foundation, 2000) and is higher in children (1–2%) than adults (less than 1%). These figures have been confirmed by double-blind, placebo-controlled, food challenges. However, the perceived incidence among adults is over 20%. The prevalence is at its highest in very young children, at 5–7%, although 80–90% of sufferers have outgrown their sensitivity by the age of 3 years. Children are particularly likely to outgrow an allergy to milk or eggs (within 12–24 months of developing it), but are less likely to outgrow allergy to peanuts or fish.

Q4.26 How are allergies and more general food intolerance diagnosed?

Food allergy is extremely difficult to diagnose; incorrect diagnosis can do more harm than good, e.g. some commercial laboratory tests of blood or hair are of dubious value. Their use may result in the inappropriate prescription of an arduous, or even nutritionally harmful, diet for a patient who does not have a food allergy at all.

Food allergy can be detected by skin tests using an extract containing the appropriate antigen (allergen) or by laboratory tests (radioallergosorbent test, commonly known as RAST). These tests are also widely used in the diagnosis of allergic disease that is not related to food. The results are likely to be positive in cases of immediate (IgE-mediated) reactions to food, but general use of these tests in the diagnosis of food allergy is controversial as a result of the difficulties in obtaining pure food proteins for testing and the consequent incidence of frequent false-positive responses. Confirmation of the existence of an allergy can be made by use of an exclusion diet, but these should be attempted only under the supervision of a dietitian. Exclusion diets involve avoidance of the suspect food in the diet until the symptoms subside. Diagnosis hinges on evidence that the symptoms return after the food is eaten again. A psychological reaction is eliminated by the investigator using a number of challenges, feeding the suspect food or a placebo (dummy treatment), where neither the investigator nor the patient knows which is which until after the test. Patients who have had severe reactions do not need to be challenged.

For the person who has had a bad experience after eating a specific food, a personal decision to eat no more of that food may do no direct harm, even if the diagnosis is wrong. However, an incorrect self-diagnosis or private diagnosis, particularly if this involves a number of foods (especially staple foods), can lead to a seriously restricted diet. It may also result in unpleasant symptoms that are related to anxiety (connected with the perpetual vigilance about diet) rather than having anything to do with the existence of a food allergy or genuine intolerance. The unnecessary avoidance of wheat can be particularly detrimental to health, because it is an important and nutritious staple in the British diet. As well as the obvious sources such as bread, pasta and breakfast cereals, wheat is used as a thickener in many other foods such as soups and sauces. In the UK, statutory fortification of wheat makes it an important source of calcium, iron, niacin and thiamin, and it makes a large contribution to the dietary intakes of these nutrients.

For tailor-made nutrition advice concerning avoidance of food allergy or any other nutrition-related disorder, such as iron-deficiency anaemia, clients should always be referred to a state-registered dietitian so that the individual's diet can be assessed and appropriate advice given on replacement foods. If diagnosis of a food allergy has been established, avoidance of the food is the mainstay of treatment, combined with other medical treatment for associated symptoms.

Q4.27 What are the problems associated with the dietary management of allergy?

Diets should not be restricted without good cause and any exclusion diet should be followed only for as long as is necessary to make or exclude a diagnosis.

The mainstay of dietetic treatment of food allergy and intolerance is the avoidance of the foods or food ingredients involved. The strictness of avoidance required depends on the severity of the reaction. The main problem that can occur is where nutritionally important staple foods need to be avoided; great care is then needed to ensure nutritional adequacy, which usually involves the provision of clear and practical advice from a dietitian. For those with severe allergic reactions (anaphylaxis), training in self-treatment (e.g. with epinephrine [adrenaline]) is useful in case of accidental exposure. Children should be given a Medic Alert symbol and, if exposure does occur, it should be treated immediately with epinephrine from a pre-loaded syringe. For some allergic conditions, there are 'free-from' lists produced by manufacturers and retailers, which can be helpful in identifying which manufactured foods needs to be avoided. The safest approach is always to check the ingredients list on the label.

Q4.28 Should women who are pregnant or breast-feeding follow special diets to reduce the risk of their child developing an allergy?

There have been suggestions that maternal avoidance (during pregnancy and lactation) of allergenic foods be used as a preventive measure for reducing the risk of allergy developing in infants. Unless there is a strong family history of allergic disease, evidence of avoidance of allergenic foods as a general preventive measure is not convincing. Indeed, it has been suggested that exposure *in utero* and via breast milk is important in establishing a normal immune response to these foods, i.e. developing tolerance to environmental proteins (see Q3.9 and Q3.10).

Q4.29 Do children grow out of their allergies?

This tends to depend on the type of allergy involved. Allergy to peanuts, for example, tends to be more severe and it is less likely that children will outgrow this type. On the other hand, children with an allergy to cows' milk or eggs are much more likely to grow out of this as they get older. It has been estimated that between 45% and 50% of infants with symptoms of cows' milk protein allergy recover by the time they are aged 1 year, 60–75% by 2 years and 85–90% by 3 years (Høst, 1997). This highlights the importance of constant monitoring, to ensure that nutritious foods are not being excluded from the diet unnecessarily. Allergic reactions to food rarely develop for the first time in adulthood.

Q4.30 What is the advice for children allergic to cows' milk?

Once an appropriate positive diagnosis has been established, cows' milk protein needs to be completely excluded from the diet. This means that, as well as excluding milk itself, all other dairy products also need to be excluded, e.g. yoghurt, fromage frais, butter and cheese. Furthermore, less obvious sources of cows' milk protein, such as products containing casein or whey (Table 4.2), also have to be removed from the diet. Clearly this can be a major undertaking.

Table 4.2 Foods containing cows' milk protein

Foods to be excluded in cows' milk protein intolerance
Soya cheese
Vegetarian cheese
Margarine and low fat spreads
Some bread
Biscuits
Sausages
Rusks
Non-milk-fat ice cream
Instant mashed potato
Muesli and other breakfast cereals
Packet and canned soups
Fish fingers and fish in batter

Infants on a cows' milk protein-free diet require a cows' milk substitute such as a special infant formula made using hydrolysed casein or whey. Advice on the most appropriate substitute should be sought from a state-registered dietitian, who will also be able to provide parents with detailed dietary advice (see Chapter 6, Q6.3).

Q4.31 Is soya milk or goats' milk a suitable alternative to cows' milk?

A soya-based formula is sometimes suggested as a replacement for cows' milk. However, many children who react adversely to cows' milk protein react in a similar way to soya protein (Høst, 1997). Indeed, it has been reported in some studies that children fed soya formula actually had the same incidence of wheezing, asthma, eczema and allergic rhinitis as children who had received cows' milk formula.

Children allergic to cows' milk are often also found to be intolerant of goats' and sheep's milk, because the proteins in all these milks are antigenically similar. Furthermore, such milks are not suitable for babies because:

- they have a high solute content;
- in an unmodified form, they are unsuitable for infants under 12 months of age;
- production of goats' milk and sheep's milk is not subjected to the same stringent hygiene regulations as cows' milk and so they carry an increased risk of gastrointestinal infection;
- the amount of some B vitamins, especially folate in goats' milk, is low.

Q4.32 Will diets that exclude key foods such as milk or wheat affect a child's growth or development?

Where foods are excluded from a child's diet, it is important to plan the diet carefully to avoid any nutritional deficiencies, which could affect growth and development. As cows' milk and its products are the major sources of calcium in the diet, complete withdrawal of such foods without compensatory replacement by other sources of calcium will mean an inadequate intake. Avoidance of wheat leads to the exclusion of many products from the diet, e.g. bread, cakes, pasta and breakfast cereals. Careful planning will be needed to ensure that suitable replacement foods are included in the diet. Exclusion of such foods in childhood should not be taken lightly and should not be attempted unless strictly necessary.

Q4.33 What causes lactose intolerance?

The most common intolerance linked to the absence of an enzyme is lactose intolerance, which occurs as a result of the absence of the enzyme lactase. Before lactose can be absorbed and utilized by the body as fuel, lactose (the sugar in milk) has to be broken down into its two component sugars, glucose and galactose, by lactase. If lactase is produced in insufficient quantities, some of the lactose can pass undigested into the large intestine, causing symptoms such as diarrhoea.

Inability to digest lactose is usually inherited and is most common in Asia and parts of Africa. People of northern European descent usually produce adequate amounts of the enzyme throughout their lives. However, in areas where the drinking of milk after infancy is relatively uncommon, enzyme levels have become genetically programmed to start to fall after early childhood, and primary lactase deficiency or primary lactase non-persistence among adolescents and adults is well known. In populations genetically prone to lactase non-persistence (e.g. Asian and Chinese populations), the prevalence of lactose maldigestion is low (5%) in children under the age of 4 years, but increases with age and plateaus at about 33% at age 13 years (Rosado, 1997).

Having a low level of lactase production does not necessarily imply lactose maldigestion or lactose intolerance. Indeed, lactose tolerance can be built up through the gradual reintroduction of lactose-containing foods in progressively increasing amounts. In the UK, is it estimated that 5% of people have lactase deficiency (National Dairy Council, 1998). However, as lactose intolerance is dose dependent and most people still produce small-to-moderate quantities of lactase, only about a third of these, 1–2%, have any symptoms. The remainder are not likely to experience any ill-effects when consuming quantities of milk and milk products typical of the British diet, and so can benefit from the nutrients that these foods provide.

Q4.34 Is hyperactivity caused by food allergy?

Hyperactivity has been reported to occur in around 1–5% of children (Committee on Toxicity of Chemicals in Food, Consumer Products and the Environment, 2000). However, evidence suggesting a relationship with food intake is very limited. A diet free from artificial additives is sometimes suggested to alleviate symptoms. There are a few studies that show some form of benefit from this type of diet; however, overall there is little robust scientific support for this approach. As such, most nutritionists remain sceptical about recommending this type of regimen.

If parents are keen to exclude additives (see Q1.13), it may be useful to give a child this type of diet for a 1-month period to assess whether there is any effect. It should be borne in mind, however, that any benefits may be a result of a non-dietary factor, such as the extra attention given to the child, rather than an actual physiological effect. Advice from a state-registered dietitian is essential before embarking on any restrictive regimen to ensure that nutritional adequacy of the diet is maintained.

Q4.35 Is migraine caused by food intolerance?

Migraine can be caused by a number of factors. The most common precipitant is stress but certain foods can also trigger a reaction. Foods such as cheese, chocolate, fish, alcohol, beans and dairy produce have all been implicated in migraine.

It is thought that the vasoactive amines in some of these foods are associated with migraines. Cheese, for example, contains tyramine, dopamine is found in broad beans and octopamine is found in citrus fruit.

Dietary factors are thought to be responsible for around a quarter to a third of cases. If particular foods are responsible for the onset of migraines in a sufferer, then avoidance of these foods may be advisable, particularly during stressful periods.

Q4.36 What is coeliac disease?

Coeliac disease (sometimes referred to as gluten-sensitive enteropathy) can be defined as an intestinal disease that occurs only when the diet provides gluten and the individual is genetically susceptible.

There are two important factors necessary for the disease to occur: a genetic predisposition to the disease and the presence of gluten in the diet to trigger the condition. The gluten fractions of wheat (gliadin), rye (secalin) and barley (hordein) are known triggering factors. There is controversy over the role of oats in the condition; this is currently the subject of a great deal of research interest. The specific peptide(s) within the triggering gluten fractions is not known, nor is the manner in which the peptide(s) triggers the abnormality. Although there are other theories, it is widely thought that the implicated gluten peptide(s) precipitates an inappropriate immune response within the gut mucosa, causing the characteristic damage. However, this particular type of immune reaction does not include the production of immunoglobulins (see Q4.29–4.33).

The lining of the small intestine, the gut mucosa (the part of the gut affected by the disease), consists of villi. These tiny finger-like projections normally provide a very large absorptive surface. A characteristic of coeliac disease is varying degrees of stunting of the small intestinal villi. This stunting causes a reduced capacity to take up nutrients provided by foods, and leads classically to diarrhoea and malnutrition.

Resolution of the symptoms and restoration of normal growth follow the removal of gluten from the diet. Later, reintroduction of gluten leads to a return of the mucosal abnormality in most cases and to clinical relapse in many but not all sufferers. The severity and timing of both are variable. About 5% (1 in 20) of children initially considered to have coeliac disease on the basis of clinical, biopsy and gluten response evidence appear to develop permanent tolerance to gluten (i.e. recover), although mucosal relapse may occur years after the reintroduction of gluten in a minority of subjects (see British Nutrition Foundation, 2000).

Q4.37 What are the main symptoms of coeliac disease?

Children diagnosed as having coeliac disease often present with failure to thrive, diarrhoea and muscle wasting, because their ability to absorb nutrients is grossly impaired. Symptoms in adults are often less acute. General tiredness and diarrhoea are common symptoms in around 80% of adults with coeliac disease. Weight loss is also common. Iron and/or folate deficiencies are frequent findings, although, in a minority of subjects, vitamin D or K is deficient. Reduced fertility and psychological disturbances are rarer findings. There is a large variation in the presentation of the disease. A patient may be severely ill, although subclinical and silent forms of the disease are also known, and these may come to light only during family or population screening. There may be a delay of several years before a correct diagnosis is reached, particularly if a patient has no weight loss or gastrointestinal symptoms.

Q4.38 What is the prevalence of coeliac disease?

Coeliac disease has been principally described in white-skinned people. Older literature suggests a prevalence of 1:1500 in the UK.

The advent of sensitive serological screening tests has, however, resulted in the suggestion that the true prevalence is greater, although many cases are mild and go undiagnosed. Studies conducted in Italy (Catassi et al., 1994) and the USA (Not et al., 1998) have investigated underlying prevalence rates (diagnosed and undiagnosed cases combined) and shown these to be around 1 in 300. A recent study in Ireland (Johnston et al., 1998) suggested a prevalence of 1 in 120.

Q4.39 How is coeliac disease diagnosed?

The 'gold standard' for diagnosis requires a biopsy in which a small piece of the small intestine is removed and examined. However, a number of blood-screening tests are now available. These detect specific antibodies associated with the presence of coeliac disease and may be used to select individuals for small intestinal biopsy from 'at-risk' groups, such as relatives of patients with the disease, or to add weight to the diagnosis. After a case of coeliac disease is diagnosed, siblings are checked for clinical history and growth rate. Any individual with a first-degree relative with coeliac disease has a 10% chance of having the condition, and should be antibody screened if there is any suspicion of the disease. It is vital that the subject is taking a gluten-containing diet either when being screened for antibodies or when having a biopsy. Those individuals who 'self-treat' or put their children onto a gluten-restricted diet before diagnosis risk getting false-negative or equivocal results, leading to a lengthy diagnostic process.

Q4.40 What is the dietary advice for people with coeliac disease?

To avoid the long-term complications of the disease, coeliac disease patients must follow a strict gluten-free diet. The risks associated with non-compliance with the diet are serious. The UK Coeliac Society publishes a yearly updated list of gluten-free foods, which it produces on the basis of information provided by food manufacturers. Patients must exercise constant vigilance when selecting processed foods because of the likelihood of wheat being present. Some gluten-free foods are available on prescription.

Wheat is widely present in foods, so a gluten-free diet, out of necessity, is quite restrictive and can be unpalatable and socially difficult to follow. Furthermore, wheat is nutritionally very important in the UK diet and its exclusion should never be considered lightly or recommended casually, unless coeliac disease has been properly diagnosed. Such patients require the expert advice of a state-registered dietitian. Token gestures, such as avoidance of pasta, will have no effect on true intolerance.

A number of products, especially for coeliac patients, are now available to replace prohibited breads, cakes and breakfast cereals based on wheat, rye and/or barley (or oats). These fall into two categories:

1. 'Naturally gluten-free' foods made from starches such as maize, potato or buckwheat. The products made from these do not rise on baking and therefore these starches are acceptable for cakes and biscuits, but are not so good for bread. The fibre content is low but can be supplemented with, for example, sugar beet fibre.
2. Foods made gluten-free by the removal of gluten from wheat flour, to produce wheat starch. The taste tends to be better, but, as it is gluten that gives wheat its unique baking qualities, the texture is still not as good as products baked with gluten-containing flour. The process of making a food gluten-free does not remove all gluten and there is always a residual gluten content. Although tolerated by most people with coeliac disease, a minority will continue to get symptoms when consuming products made from wheat starch. These individuals should switch to wheat-free (naturally gluten-free) products.

Implementation of a strict gluten-free diet normally leads to reversal of any nutritional deficiency without the use of supplements. However, if there has been a severe deficiency of a particular nutrient, supplementation on the advice of either a GP or state-registered dietitian may be appropriate.

For more information, contact the UK Coeliac Society (see Useful addresses).

Special Diets from the Perspective of the Community Nurse

Q4.41 Is there any special advice for people diagnosed as HIV positive?

Weight loss is a common feature of HIV infection. Wasting often begins early in the disease and becomes progressively worse. Poor nutritional status can result from several factors, including a loss of appetite, accelerated metabolism, drug/nutrient interactions and gastrointestinal disturbances. Increased metabolic needs are usually caused by acute episodes of opportunistic infection, which increase the body's requirements for protein and energy. Psychological factors also have an impact on nutritional status. Anxiety and depression are common reactions in people living with HIV and can have an adverse effect on appetite. The combined effects on the immune system of both malnutrition and HIV infection may hasten the course of the disease. For people with AIDS, malnutrition and weight loss correlate strongly with a diminished survival time. Preventing and treating malnutrition and wasting should, therefore, be a high priority in the care of HIV-infected patients. Teaching HIV-infected individuals about the importance of good diet in maintaining health and promoting the effective functioning of the immune system is likely to improve the quality and quantity of their nutrient intake. A chapter on the interrelationship between nutrition and the immune system will be found in a British Nutrition Foundation Task Force Report on Adverse Reactions to Food, due to be published in 2001.

Nutritional interventions cannot change the ultimate outcome of HIV infection but can slow its progression and improve quality of life. Good nutrition may also improve people's responses to drug therapy, reduce the length of time spent in hospital and promote physical independence. Early nutritional intervention may detect and correct subclinical deficiencies in preparation for the stresses ahead. It also provides baseline assessment parameters to assist in monitoring changes in nutrition status. Although the exact mineral and vitamin requirements for people with HIV and AIDS have not been determined, meeting at least the daily requirement for these nutrients is essential. Studies have shown that the intake of several micronutrients, including B vitamins, vitamin E and zinc, often fall below the recommended levels (Abrams et al., 1993; Tang et al., 1993; Baum et al., 1994). People who are not able to eat sufficient food to ensure that their requirements are met daily might benefit from a multivitamin and mineral supplement. Susceptibility to food-borne illness requires that individuals with HIV should be given detailed instructions about the safe handling of food (see Q5.16). The diagnosis of HIV infection should be followed by specialist nutritional/dietetic advice. However, nurses can help by identifying nutritional problems, prescribing appropriate interventions and reinforcing specialist dietetic advice.

Q4.42 Is there any special dietary advice for people with established cancer?

Cancer is often associated with severe weight loss caused by increased metabolic requirements and a loss of appetite. As soon as a diagnosis is made, a supportive diet, which is typically higher than normal in nutrient content, should be devised. Many patients require supple-mentary and tube feeding and some parenteral nutrition. Dietary modifications may be necessary as a result of ileostomy or colostomy. Although a good diet cannot cure any type of cancer, it can support the immune system and improve the comfort of patients, as well as their sense of well-being. Taste changes are associated with anorexia, and a careful evaluation of food likes and dislikes and attention to the appearance and taste of foods can make a substantial contribution to the amount of food consumed and hence help reduce weight loss.

Q4.43 Is there any special dietary advice for people who have already suffered a heart attack?

Stopping smoking, taking regular exercise and following an appro-priate diet can reduce the risk of a second heart attack. Several of the nutritional factors associated with a reduced risk of heart disease are even more important for people who have already had a heart attack (see Q4.2). For obese patients, a diet to promote weight reduction should be encouraged. Reducing fat intake, particularly saturated fatty acid intake, by selecting lean cuts of meat and lower fat dairy products; by reducing the use of oil and full-fat spreads (margarine, butter); by eating fewer fried foods; and by moderating consumption of high-fat foods such as cakes, biscuits and crisps as savoury snacks, will help to reduce blood cholesterol levels. An increase in dietary carbohydrate, primarily in the form of starches and complex carbo-hydrate, has been recommended to replace dietary fat. Eating a vari-ety of fruit and vegetables will also increase fibre intake and provide a range of antioxidant nutrients (vitamin E, vitamin C, β-carotene), which may help protect against worsening atherosclerosis. For patients with hypertension, reducing salt intake may be beneficial but increasing physical activity, stopping smoking and avoiding excessive alcohol consumption are also important.

There is evidence that a diet similar to that consumed traditionally in Mediterranean countries may be of benefit to people who have existing heart disease. The Lyon Diet Heart Study, a secondary prevention trial, found that a diet containing no butter, cream or milk, lots of vegetables, fruit, bread and cereals, and a little meat reduced deaths and cardiovascular events by over 70%, without having any effect on cholesterol levels (De Lorgeril et al., 1994). Patients used margarine made from rapeseed oil (rich in monounsaturated fatty acids and the n-3 fatty acid, α-linolenic acid) and drank wine during the study, both of which are dietary factors that might help protect against recurrent heart attacks. Although heavy alcohol consumption will increase the risk of another heart attack, alcoholic drinks need not be avoided. In fact the beneficial effect of a moderate intake is likely to be more apparent for those with one or more risk factors for heart disease or those who have already suffered a heart attack.

Secondary trials have also shown that eating oily fish or taking a fish-oil supplement can reduce the risk of a second heart attack (see British Nutrition Foundation, 1999c). A 2-year study in Wales (Burr et al., 1989) investigated 2000 men who had recently had a heart attack and found that the group advised to eat more oil-rich fish or take fish-oil capsules every day had 29% fewer deaths than those who did not change their diet. This difference was attributable to a reduction in CHD deaths. Although there were fewer fatal heart attacks in those who ate more fish, the number of non-fatal attacks remained the same. In other words, eating oil-rich fish regularly seems to reduce the risk of death, rather than preventing a second heart attack from occurring (see Q5.7). Recently, these findings were confirmed by the GISSI trial which demonstrated the same protective effect with fish-oil supplements (GISSI, 1999).

Q4.44 Which dietary considerations are important for people in the
        community on dialysis?

Patients receiving dialysis do have special dietary requirements and must be advised on an individual basis by a dietitian. In general, a high-fibre, low-fat and low-sugar diet should be recommended to limit the risk of hyperlipidaemia. Hyperlipidaemia contributes to the high incidence of heart disease among patients on haemodialysis and peritoneal dialysis. Obese dialysis patients should be encouraged to lose weight. However, this must be done under the strict supervision of a doctor or dietitian. Potassium and sodium restriction may be advised and vitamin supplements are usually prescribed (particularly folic acid and vitamin C). Iron supplements are given to make up for blood losses during haemodialysis. Calcium and phosphate levels are also regularly monitored in all patients on dialysis.

> Q4.45 Which dietary considerations are important for people in the
> community with liver disease?

Liver function can be impaired by a number of disorders and diseases, the most common of which include hepatitis and cirrhosis. Patients with mild hepatitis often suffer from nausea and a lack of appetite. Foods such as milk, butter and cheese are usually well tolerated and a diet that is generally nutritious and high in protein and energy is recommended. As bile salt production may be impaired, some patients are advised to reduce their fat intake. Vitamin supplementation may also have been recommended, particularly in cases of alcoholic hepatitis or cirrhosis.

> Q4.46 Which dietary considerations are important for people in the
> community with gastrointestinal problems, e.g. Crohn's
> disease and ulcerative colitis?

The most common gastrointestinal problem is irritable bowel syndrome (IBS). The cause of IBS is not known. Patients with IBS often expect dietary advice and frequently cite foods that they believe exacerbate their symptoms. However, dietary restriction of these foods should not be encouraged without adequate supervision because this may lead to nutritional deficiencies. Dietary intervention works for some sufferers, some of the time, but there does not seem to be a simple answer (see Q5.13).

The dietary management of Crohn's disease attempts to meet the nutritional requirements in the face of symptoms that often interfere with dietary adequacy. Nutritional problems, particularly anaemia and weight loss, are common. Dietary management is therefore aimed at improving appetite, reducing malabsorption and correcting micronutrient inadequacies associated with anaemia (iron, vitamin B_{12} and folate). Drugs can lead to the depression of appetite, but eliminating zinc deficiency is also important. For patients who do not respond to conventional treatment in Crohn's disease, various enteral and parenteral regimens may be used.

Diet has little influence in ulcerative colitis, although many patients do ask for nutritional advice. Patients should be encouraged to eat as normal a diet as possible. Some patients' symptoms may be aggravated by lactase deficiency and therefore improve on a diet free of cows' milk (see Q4.33).

Q4.47 Which dietary considerations are important for people who are underweight?

The causes of being underweight are extremely diverse but certain groups within the community, such as elderly people, are particularly vulnerable. A screening tool to identify underweight and undernutrition has been developed by the Malnutrition Advisory Group (2000) (see Useful Addresses). Patients who have anorexia nervosa may be extremely underweight and should be encouraged to seek medical advice as soon as possible (see Q3.74). To gain weight, a person must increase his or her energy intake by selecting energy-dense foods (which also provide a good range of nutrients), eating regular meals, taking larger portions and consuming extra snacks and beverages. Conventional advice is to consume around 1000 kcal above normal energy needs. High-protein and energy supplements can also be used, in addition to regular meals, to help regain weight. For people who are underweight as a result of illness, concentrated liquid formulas may be recommended because these are easy to swallow and digest. As fat contains more than twice as much energy as the same weight of carbohydrate, it adds energy without adding too much bulk. However, the consumption of a very-high-fat diet is contrary to healthy eating recommendations. Advice to increase fat intake should encourage the selection of foods rich in monunsaturated and polyunsaturated fatty acids, rather than those rich in saturated fatty acids (see Q2.4 and Table 2.1).

Q4.48 Which types of food can be recommended when there are eating or
swallowing difficulties?

A variety of different conditions can lead to eating difficulties. These
include: few or no teeth; chewing or swallowing difficulties; diseases
of the mouth, throat, oesophagus or stomach; and fractured or wired
jaws. A soft, semi-solid or liquid diet is useful for patients who are
unable to consume a normal diet. Foods can be chopped, minced or
puréed depending on individual needs. Meals should be served with
plenty of sauce or gravy to facilitate feeding and swallowing. Soups
and milk puddings are easily swallowed. Liquidised foods usually
require the addition of a substantial amount of liquid to obtain the
correct consistency. This results in a large volume that makes it difficult for patients to obtain a sufficient nutrient intake. Concentrated
energy supplements may consequently be necessary. It is therefore
essential to ensure that the diet provides sufficient energy and
micronutrients, as well as the desired consistency.

Chapter 5
Issues in the Media

Stories about diet, nutrition and health appear in newspapers, in magazines, on the radio and on television on a regular basis. Indeed, most people get most of their information about diet and health through these media. It is sometimes difficult to differentiate the myth from the fact. Some media items are well reported and contain expert quotes from reputable scientists; at the other end of the spectrum are stories based purely on fiction which are misleading, unhelpful and confusing for the public. This can sometimes be the result of a journalist taking a leap of faith when looking for a new angle: editors are less likely to use stories based on the 'good old healthy balanced diet message', and some journalists may be tempted to use information arising from novel one-off reports from fringe sources if it makes a good story.

This is part of the reason why there is a public perception that nutrition experts do not agree or regularly change their minds. Genuine nutrition experts, such as state-registered dietitians or registered public health nutritionists (see Q6.3 and Q6.4) and those engaged in research in university departments and research institutes, do in general agree on what constitutes a healthy diet and promote consistent messages over time. Of course, there will always be changes in the detail of nutrition messages, as new science emerges but, broadly speaking, messages about optimal dietary intake have remained constant for some time. For example, fruit and vegetables are universally recommended these days, but their importance was also acknowledged during the war years when we were advised to 'dig for victory'.

When a new story is promoted by the media, the best course of action is to look at the original research paper and evaluate it critically (see Q6.1 and Q6.2). It will then be possible to establish the validity of the story and formulate appropriate advice. It may also be helpful to look at the credentials of the 'experts' quoted, or interviewed, as part of the story to ascertain their level of credibility.

Some of the popular press stories that have appeared recently are listed below.

Dieting and Weight Loss

As the number of obese and overweight people in this country continues to increase, issues around diet and weight loss regularly appear in the media. This is likely to continue into the future.

Q5.1 Are there any miracle diets?

It seems that not a day goes by without some new 'miracle' diet being promoted in newspapers, in magazines or in bookshops – most offer drastic weight loss without the need for any effort. Unfortunately, there is no such thing as a 'miracle' weight-loss cure. People who promote such regimens are at best misguided and at worst unscrupulous charlatans exploiting those who are desperate to lose weight, at any cost.

The energy balance equation is one of the few statements about obesity that can be made with absolute certainty. Energy intake minus energy expenditure equals change in body energy stores. In other words, weight loss will not occur unless the amount of energy used by the body exceeds the amount being consumed via food and drink. This is worth remembering when a diet plan suggests that weight loss can occur in the absence of any change to dietary habits or lifestyle.

For those who wish to lose weight, advice should be to forget the miracle cures – they do not work. Instead, a sensible approach to weight loss should be promoted. There are two main ways of achieving this:

1. Eating less or exercising more
2. A combination of the two.

For people with just a few pounds to lose, probably the best approach is to be more physically active. This will help relaxation and will benefit the heart, bones and digestive system. It does not have to mean taking up a sport or religiously attending aerobics classes – although this is a good idea. It can be as simple as walking to the shops rather than taking the bus or car, using stairs rather than the lift, or going for a long walk or cycle ride at the weekend with friends or family. By choosing types of activity that focus on the muscles in the area where the unwanted fat is deposited, you can help tone the muscles and improve the general appearance of the target region.

Frequent dieting can take the enjoyment out of eating and crash diets may do more harm than good. Although crash diets do result in rapid weight loss, much of this loss will be lean body tissue. As soon as normal eating is re-established, weight will pile back on.

A sensible weight loss is 1–2 lb per week and this should be achievable if people stick to a balanced diet that provides plenty of fruit and vegetables, incorporates lean meat, chicken, fish, pulses and low-fat dairy products, and which has plenty of starchy foods such as pasta, rice, potatoes and bread. Yes, these are an important part of a healthy slimming diet, provided that they are not accompanied by lots of spread, oil or rich sauces. The easiest way of eating fewer calories is to cut down on fatty foods because dietary fat provides more calories, weight for weight, than starch, sugar or protein. Another useful way is to cut down consumption of alcoholic drinks.

To keep trim, rather than spending money on slimming aids that offer miracle cures, patients/clients might be better advised to invest in an annual membership of their local leisure centre or gym, or to buy a second-hand bicycle and put it to good use.

Q5.2 What are the health implications of yo-yo dieting?

'Yo-yo dieting' is a term sometimes used to describe the pattern of repeated losses and subsequent regain of body weight experienced by some women who spend much of their life 'dieting'. This sort of pattern is also known as weight cycling, and is not confined to people who are overweight.

It is now clear that, when we lose weight, there is a fall in our basal metabolic rate (BMR) – the amount of energy (calories) we need to go about our day-to-day lives. This is because the BMR is related to the amount of lean tissue (e.g. muscle) we have. When we lose weight, most of the loss is fat or adipose tissue, but a proportion of the loss is non-fat tissue. Furthermore, the relative amount of lean tissue lost is greater when weight loss is very rapid. This is why experts recommend a gradual weight loss of about 2 lb (1 kg) per week on an energy intake of about 1500 kcal/day (6.3 MJ/day) for women, combined with an increase in physical activity. When weight is regained, the BMR increases. Consequently, heavier people typically need slightly more food energy to maintain their body weight than very slim people.

Although being obese is not beneficial to health, some concern has been expressed about the potential negative health consequences of yo-yo dieting.

The majority of long-term studies into the health risks of yo-yo dieting or weight cycling show that men and women undergoing body weight fluctuations are at higher risk of early death and cardiovascular disease. No studies show that weight fluctuation is beneficial. However, the precise role of dieting is unclear.

This situation should not be used as an excuse for not tackling that spare tyre. Two of the largest studies both suggest that any adverse effects of weight fluctuation occur in relatively normal weight subjects rather than in those tackling a genuine weight problem (British Nutrition Foundation, 1999a).

The messages from this research are that people who are not overweight should be encouraged to maintain a normal weight rather than a fashionably underweight state. Also, more attention should be paid to helping overweight people maintain their weight loss, rather than falling into a loss–regain–loss cycle.

Q5.3 What causes cellulite?

Cellulite is nothing more than a trendy name for fat that becomes dimpled because of where it is deposited. Nutritionists are often asked whether there is a magic diet that will selectively slim down the hips or thighs. Of course, the answer is no – the body does not work that way. But these problem areas can be tackled by being selective in the way physical activity is used to keep in trim.

Even the slimmest of people have a certain amount of fat distributed around their bodies; healthy slim women typically have about

20–25% of their body weight as fat. For men, the figure is a little lower. This fat is typically stored around the hips or the waist, and to a large extent this distribution is genetically determined and varies with gender. These stores serve a variety of very useful purposes. The fat cushions body organs such as the kidneys, it helps us to keep warm and it acts as an energy store.

Nevertheless, one can have too much of a good thing and over half the adult population is now recognised to be overweight (see Q3.81). Some people will go to any lengths to find a quick and pain-less solution to those unwanted pounds. But the facts of the matter are that there are no quick and simple answers. There are no 'wonder' foods or supplements that can cause the pounds to fall off all by themselves. Nor can slimming diets cause weight loss from a particular part of the body.

Forget the 'magic' creams, potions and pills that claim to dissolve cellulite; the only way to lose excess fat – including cellulite – is to ensure that the amount of energy (calories) expended is more than the amount of energy provided by the foods and drinks eaten. There are no ways of getting round the basic laws of physics.

Women's Issues

Issues that relate to women's health and well-being, such as premen-strual syndrome and the menopause, represent another area that is often the subject of media interest. In particular, the possible role of diet and nutrition in alleviating symptoms is frequently discussed.

> Q5.4 Which dietary factors can help to alleviate the symptoms of premenstrual syndrome?

Premenstrual syndrome (PMS) describes a range of symptoms that some women experience between the middle and the end (luteal phase) of a menstrual cycle. The most frequently reported discom-forts include water retention, irritability, depression, backache and breast tenderness. These usually disappear soon after menstruation begins.

Attempts to identify physiological factors to explain why some women have PMS have failed, because hormone levels and patterns of fluctuation have repeatedly been shown to be no different to those in women who report never experiencing PMS.

Several aspects of diet have been considered, but as yet there is no clear evidence for a role of any specific dietary component.

It has been suggested that a fall in the production of substances known as neurotransmitters may lead to changes in mood. It is known that vitamin B_6 is needed in the synthesis of some neurotransmitters, e.g. serotonin and dopamine, and it has therefore been suggested that vitamin B_6 supplements might be of help (Gaby et al., 1991). One of the few well-controlled trials examining this claim indicated a possible improvement of symptoms, but gave no evidence of potent effects of supplements of the vitamin (50 mg/day was used in the trial) (Doll et al., 1989).

It has been recognised for some time that high doses of vitamin B_6 can result in damage to the peripheral nervous system if taken over a long period of time. As many women have been taking vitamin B_6 supplements in the hope that they might alleviate symptoms of PMS, the Government recently asked the Food Advisory Committee (FAC) to consider the safety of supplements and, in particular, the level at which toxicity symptoms might be expected to occur. The Government's Committee on Toxicity of Chemicals in Food, Consumer Products and the Environment (COT) provided detailed advice on the toxicity of vitamin B_6 (Committee on Toxicity, 1997).

As a result of the advice they received, in 1998 the Government proposed the need for legislation to limit the availability of vitamin B_6 supplements. The proposal was that only products containing up to 10 mg/tablet would be available freely, and all supplements containing vitamin B_6 should carry a warning label about the risk of harmful effects of higher intakes over 10 mg/day. It was also proposed that products containing up to 49 mg of vitamin B_6 per tablet must be sold under the control and supervision of a pharmacist, and doses of 50 mg upwards would be available only on medical prescription. Subsequently, it was decided to delay further pronouncements until the special Expert Group on Vitamins and Minerals, set up by the Government, had presented its findings on vitamin and mineral safety. The findings of this committee (likely to be available in 2001) are awaited before new legislation is considered.

Several minerals, e.g. zinc and magnesium, are also involved in the production of neurotransmitters in the body and they have been studied in relation to PMS. Again, there is no convincing evidence of any benefit of supplements.

There has also been interest in a particular fatty acid, GLA (γ-linoleic acid), found in evening primrose oil. Some women report relief from symptoms when they take GLA but others perceive no benefit. Clearly more research is needed in this area.

To sum up, it is unclear why some women suffer from PMS. The involvement of dietary factors is to a large extent speculative, but a number of threads of evidence are appearing, which may help make the picture clearer and be of benefit to women.

Q5.5 What dietary factors are important during the menopause?

Articles frequently appear in the press aimed at women of menopausal age. During the menopause, as with any other time in life, it is important to aim for a varied and well-balanced diet which will help ensure optimal nutritional intake and status (see Q1.6). For those watching their weight, the dietary messages remain the same, although advice should be to cut down a little more on the amounts of food eaten, and in particular to watch fat and alcohol intake – these are concentrated sources of calories. There are no miracle cures for weight loss (see Q5.1); sensible eating and gentle regular exercise are by far the best long-term solutions to the problem.

There are also some specific nutritional issues that may be of interest. Intake of a number of nutrients, including calcium and vitamin D, is important, along with physical activity, to help ensure optimal bone health (see Q3.99). Iron requirements fall slightly when menstruation stops.

The role of calcium in the prevention of bone mineral loss during the menopause has been studied extensively. Calcium supplementation does not seem to have any major effect on bone mineral density at the time of the menopause. However, studies on women 5 years after the menopause are more positive and show a slower loss of bone with calcium supplementation (Department of Health, 1998a). More research is needed in this area. At present, advice should be to include a range of good sources of calcium in the diet to ensure optimal intake (see Q3.98).

Body levels of vitamin D are also known to be important (see Q2.22).

We should all aim for 30 minutes of physical activity at least five times a week to ensure that we stay fit and healthy and to help maintain a sensible body weight (see Q3.87). This can also help to maintain bone strength and sense of well-being.

Iron deficiency and low iron stores are a significant problem for many women of child-bearing age, particularly in those who have heavy periods and/or poor dietary intakes of iron. At the time of the menopause, when periods stop, the iron recommendations for women are reduced to the same level as those for men (8.7 mg/day) (see Table 1.3). Even though iron requirements are not as high in postmenopausal women, it is still important to include a range of iron-containing foods in the diet (see Q2.6).

There has been much interest in recent months in the possible role of phyto-oestrogens in the alleviation of menopausal symptoms, particularly hot flushes and vaginitis (see Q3.99). The prevalence of these symptoms is much lower in Japanese women than in women in Western countries, and it has been suggested that this is a result of our lower intake of phyto-oestrogens. Hormone replacement therapy (HRT) generally alleviates these symptoms, but many people are looking for a more natural alternative.

Several studies have looked at the effect of phyto-oestrogens on the symptoms of the menopause. Some have shown a beneficial effect and others have shown no effect (Cassidy et al., 1994). Further studies are needed in this area before firm recommendations and advice can be given. For those who wish to try increasing their intake of phyto-oestrogens, the main sources are linseed, soyabeans, tofu, soyabean flour and soya milk, although many plant foods contain small amounts (see Q3.99).

Functional Foods

Q5.6 What are functional foods?

Functional foods first emerged in Japan, where many products are now available (see Buttriss, 2000a).

A functional ingredient can be defined as: 'a dietary ingredient that affects its host in a targeted manner so as to exert positive effects that may, in due course, justify certain health claims.' In other words, foods containing these ingredients (functional foods) are foods that have health-promoting properties over and above their nutritional value (see Q1.16).

The term 'functional foods' can be viewed as encompassing a very broad range of products, ranging from foods generated around a particular functional ingredient (e.g. plant stanol-enriched spreads), through to staple everyday foods fortified with a nutrient that would not usually be present to any great extent (e.g. folic acid-fortified bread or breakfast cereals). Also encompassed within the range are foods providing probiotic bacteria, e.g. types of yoghurts and other fermented milk products, and prebiotics, which are substances that promote growth of specific bacteria, e.g. oligosaccharides such as inulin (see Q1.17).

It is important to assess each individual food on its own merit. In particular, it is crucial that solid science exists to underpin the claims being made. Ideally this should include evidence that the substance is absorbed or reaches its site of action, that consumption of the food beneficially influences a physiological function (e.g. blood pressure) or a biomarker recognised to have an impact on health (e.g. blood cholesterol) and, ideally, that this effect has a direct impact on health status.

The level of consumption of the food that is required to achieve a beneficial effect on health is also an important consideration. In particular, it should be possible to achieve the required level of intake of the functional food or ingredient within normal dietary patterns.

Functional foods may provide benefits in health terms, but should not be seen as an alternative to a varied and balanced diet and a healthy lifestyle. To maximise health and well-being, people should be encouraged to avoid smoking, take plenty of exercise and have a varied diet, which is low in fat and includes plenty of fruit and vegetables. Functional foods will not be a miracle solution to health problems, but may be useful to some people as part of a healthy diet and lifestyle.

A possible disadvantage of functional foods, from a health education point of view, is that they may obscure the boundaries between food groups (normally defined by the specific selection of nutrients that foods in each group provide). This inevitably influences the ease with which simple and practical dietary advice can be formulated.

Currently, food law does not specifically encompass claims about health-promoting properties of functional foods. However, it is generally accepted that 'health-promoting' claims (e.g. 'helps lower blood cholesterol when consumed as part of a low-fat diet') rather than 'disease prevention or medical' claims (e.g. helps prevent heart disease) can be made provided that the claim is underpinned by sound science and is not misleading. The relevant food law that identifies the boundaries for such claims is embodied in the Food Safety Act 1990, which states that claims must not mislead the consumer as to the nature or quality of a food, and the Food Labelling Regulations 1996 which allow declaration of the nutrient content of foods and claims such as 'low fat' or 'high fibre', but prohibit medicinal claims such as ' prevents' or 'treats' or 'cures' a disease.

In the absence of specific legislation, several initiatives are under way to provide guidance on the type of evidence required to support claims, the nature of claims that might be acceptable and a voluntary code to be followed by those making claims, for example the Joint Health Claims Initiative launched in December 2000 (see Useful Addresses).

Some examples of functional foods recently launched on to the market include eggs enriched with n-3 fatty acids and spreads with plant stanol or sterol esters (see Q5.8).

Q5.7 What are the health benefits of n-3 fatty acids?

It is known that long-chain n-3 (or ω-3) fatty acids reduce the risk of suffering a fatal heart attack and have an important role in maintaining heart health. These n-3 fatty acids are provided in abundance in fish oils, and they are also present in the flesh of oil-rich fish, such as mackerel, salmon, kippers, herrings, sprats, trout, sardines and pilchards. They can also be manufactured in the body from the shorter-chain n-3 fatty acid, α-linolenic acid, an essential fatty acid found in green vegetables and seeds such as linseed. In 1994, the Government's advisory committee COMA (Department of Health, 1994b) recommended that people eat at least two portions of fish a week, one of which should be oil-rich fish. This is advice for the general population but, for people who have already suffered a heart attack, there is good evidence that 400 g oil-rich fish per week can reduce the chance of a second attack (see British Nutrition Foundation, 1999c). Currently, only about a third of adults eat any oil-rich fish and current consumers typically have the equivalent of one small serving (135 g) per week. Given current preferences, therefore, it may be that for many people this advice is not a readily accepted means of consuming n-3 fatty acids.

Recently, eggs enriched with *n*-3 fatty acids were launched in the UK. Substitution of standard eggs by these *n*-3-enriched eggs provides an alternative and practical source of *n*-3 fatty acids, for those who do not wish to consume more oil-rich fish.

Consumption of three to four eggs per week would provide the same amount of *n*-3 fatty acids as recommended in the COMA report on Nutritional Aspects of Cardiovascular Disease (Department of Health, 1994b), although the cost of these eggs is around 10 pence more than the standard price for eggs per half dozen.

Q5.8 What are plant stanol or sterol esters?

A new range of fat and cheese spreads was launched in March 1999 under the brand name Benecol. Subsequently, later in the year a similar product (Flora Proactiv) was launched by Unilever. These products contain cholesterol-like substances found in plants, plant stanol or plant sterol esters, which have cholesterol-lowering properties. Plant stanols and plant sterols are related to naturally occurring substances found in many grains, such as wheat, rye and maize, and usually are present in the diet in small amounts.

Plant stanols have a similar structure to cholesterol and so have the ability to inhibit the absorption of cholesterol in the gut. The cholesterol present in the intestine comes from three sources: the diet, which contributes 300–400 mg/day in the average adult; the bile, which contributes 750–1250 mg (which is usually available for re-absorption); and the cells of the gut wall, the contribution of which is small.

These products may be helpful for those with raised blood cholesterol levels, if the product is substituted for a standard product and eaten as part of a cholesterol-lowering diet and in conjunction with a healthy lifestyle. However, it is important to recognise that such products address only one risk factor for coronary heart disease, which is a multifactorial disease. They are not a magic solution and should not be considered an alternative to a healthy balanced diet or a healthy lifestyle. Probably the most effective ways of reducing heart disease risk are to give up smoking and to be more physically active.

These products are also relatively expensive, and may be out of the reach of those in society with the highest prevalence of heart disease – low-income groups (see Q3.103–3.108).

A number of other aspects of diet are also important. Antioxidant nutrients, found in a variety of foods, and some plant substances such as flavonoids (see Q5.9), that also have antioxidant properties, may reduce risk from CHD (see Q4.2). Therefore, it is important to increase intake of fruit and vegetables to at least five portions per day. Fruit and vegetables, and also beans, pulses and some grains (e.g. oats), contain soluble fibre which may help lower blood cholesterol levels. In addition, the oils found in oil-rich fish have been shown to have a beneficial effect on different factors in the blood and may be effective in reducing risk (see Q5.7). It is also important to cut down on fat, particularly sources of saturated fatty acids, by, for example, selecting leaner cuts of meat and lower-fat dairy products, and reducing intake of fried foods, pastries and biscuits. In other words, the dietary message is one of balance and variety.

Protective Substances in Food and Their Impact on Health

There is a great deal of media interest in the various potentially protective substances found in foods, sometimes referred to as phyto-chemicals or plant chemicals, and their role in promoting optimal health (see Q2.9 and Q4.2). This is an interesting area of emerging science and is a subject currently being reviewed by an expert Task Force set up in July 1999 by the British Nutrition Foundation. The findings of this Task Force will be published in 2001 in a comprehensive new report. It is a good example of how emerging science has identified the fact that components of foods, which have not formerly been recognised as nutrients, may in fact be important for health.

Q5.9 How can flavonoids affect health?

It is well known that fruit and vegetables are essential foods in a healthy diet, but the search is still on for the precise reason for this. It was initially assumed that the substances responsible for the health-promoting properties were vitamins, such as vitamin C and β-carotene. We now know that, although these remain important, this is just part of the picture.

Important new research is now identifying a whole host of plant substances that appear to have beneficial properties, at least in animal and *in vitro* studies These can be found in a range of foods, including onions, lettuce, tomatoes, brussel sprouts, tea and red wine. The research shows that even for a particular type of food, depending on the variety, the phytochemical content can vary considerably.

This adds a new dimension to the five-a-day fruit and vegetable message. Not only do we need to think about five different fruit and vegetables each day, in the future we may even be in a position to make our selection armed with knowledge of how individual varieties fare in the league table for phytochemical content.

Q5.10 What is the role of phyto-oestrogens in health?

Phyto-oestrogens (principally isoflavones and lignans) are plant-derived substances that have both oestrogenic and antioestrogenic effects. They compete with natural oestradiol to bind with the oestrogen receptor complex. However, on binding, they fail to stimulate a full oestrogenic response.

Phyto-oestrogens are found in a number of plants, but the richest source is soya beans (see Q3.99). It has been proposed that phyto-oestrogens may offer some protection against a wide range of conditions, including breast, bowel, prostate and other cancers. Despite a plausible mechanism, however, there is little observational evidence for a protective effect against cancer. Protection has also been proposed for cardiovascular disease and menopausal symptoms (Cassidy et al., 1994).

It has been suggested that symptoms of the menopause and incidence of osteoporosis in menopausal women may be reduced through the oestrogenic properties of the phyto-oestrogens (see Q3.99).

Concerns have been expressed over the long-term effects of phyto-oestrogens given to infants and young children via soya formula. Currently, breast milk or cows' milk formula is recommended for infant feeding, unless there is a clear indication that soya milk formula is required on medical grounds. It should be noted that infants allergic to cows' milk are, in around 5–10% of cases, also at risk of developing allergy to soya (MacDonald, 1995) (see Q4.31).

The role of phyto-oestrogens in health is one of the topics being addressed by a British Nutrition Foundation Task Force reviewing the data about protective factors in plants. The Task Force's Report is due to be published in 2001.

Q5.11 How can tomatoes and lycopene protect against disease?

Recent press interest has focused on the suggestion that lycopene can provide protection against oxidative damage, reducing risk of cancer and coronary heart disease.

Lycopene is a carotenoid. Unlike β-carotene it cannot be converted to vitamin A in the body, but it is a potent antioxidant (see Q2.8). The main sources of lycopene in the British diet are tomatoes and tomato products, although some is present in watermelon, pink grapefruit and canned apricots. Food processing increases the availability of lycopene, so more is present in canned and puréed tomatoes than in fresh ones. Lycopene may be a marker of certain types of dietary behaviour, so we should be cautious about taking cocktails of dietary supplements. The main carotenoids in adipose tissue are β-carotene, α-carotene and lycopene.

It has been suggested that lycopene is protective against prostate cancer, because it is found to be actively concentrated in prostate tissue (Department of Health, 1998c). Observational studies have shown that tomato consumption is associated with a reduced risk of prostate cancer. It has also been suggested that lycopene consumption is associated with reduced risk of breast, colon, stomach and lung cancers. To date, however, although there is epidemiological evidence of a beneficial effect there have been no placebo-controlled intervention trials in humans. This would be needed before health claims could be made. The best advice at present is to incorporate into the diet a wide variety of fruit and vegetables, including tomatoes and other sources of lycopene.

Q5.12 What is the role of diet in osteoporosis?

Osteoporosis is a complex disease that is affected by a number of factors, including race, genetics and physical and cultural factors. It is a disease characterised by loss of bone mass and increased risk of bone fracture. It is not primarily a nutritional disease, although appropriate nutritional intake, along with regular weight-bearing physical activity, can have an impact on bone health and can help to prevent osteoporosis. Osteoporosis is commonly associated with postmenopausal women. It can also occur in other age groups, e.g. children and young adults, in pregnant women (although this is relatively rare), in men and secondary to conditions such as anorexia nervosa or those that require long-term use of steroids.

The future impact of osteoporosis is likely to be far reaching as the number of older people in the population increases. Recent estimates suggest that the cost to the NHS of this disease has now risen to £942 million per annum (Department of Health, 1998a). Strategies need to be implemented to optimise bone health and so reduce incidence of this disease in the future.

Recommendations have been published recently by the Department of Health in a recent COMA Report on the nutritional aspects of bone health (Department of Health, 1998a). A healthy lifestyle to maintain bone health should be encouraged at all ages. A varied diet combined with regular weight-bearing physical activity is the best way forward. Dietary means of achieving an adequate calcium intake should be encouraged (see Q2.5).

Vitamin D was also highlighted in the Report as an important nutrient in relation to bone health. It was recommended that the public and health professionals should be better informed about the importance of achieving adequate vitamin D status (see Q2.22), particularly as there is recent evidence (Finch et al., 1998) that the vitamin D status of many people over the age of 65 years is relatively poor (see Q3.79, Q3.109 and Q3.113). For further information, see Q4.15.

Q5.13 What is the role of diet in irritable bowel syndrome?

Irritable bowel syndrome (IBS) is a very common but poorly understood disorder in which there are often extreme responses to stimuli such as specific foods, stress and distension (Edwards, 1996). It has been suggested that about half of the people attending gastroenterology clinics have IBS. The symptoms are abdominal pain and discomfort, and an alteration in bowel habit, which may be either constipation or diarrhoea. The pain is usually related to either meals or defecation. These symptoms can also be features of other bowel disorders and so IBS is often diagnosed by a process of elimination. Other symptoms, not involving the large bowel, can also be present.

It is generally agreed that there are subgroups of patients with different sets of symptoms and different underlying causes, e.g. stress, hyperventilation and air swallowing, and hormonal factors. Effective therapy is likely to result from identification of these subgroups, e.g.

those with the symptomatic extremes of predominately constipation or predominately diarrhoea, although this is made more complicated by the fact that patients can fluctuate between the two extremes. In two patients, similar symptoms might have very different causes and so a treatment that works for the one may not work for the other.

A high-fibre diet, with or without bran supplements, is commonly prescribed to treat IBS, despite the lack of agreement on the benefits of this form of treatment. A recent review of studies focusing on a high-fibre or bran-supplemented diet showed a significant improvement in symptoms in only two of the eight studies (Rees et al., 1994). IBS patients who suffer with constipation are highly likely to experience relief of symptoms if they increase their intake of dietary fibre. However, such a diet may exacerbate symptoms such as distension, flatulence, diarrhoea and abdominal pain.

Some IBS patients associate their symptoms with eating particular types of food. But there is no real evidence to suggest that specific exclusion diets are routinely beneficial. Indeed, eliminating key foods, and consequently unbalancing the diet, can sometimes do more harm than good. If such diets are to be tried, they should be under medical supervision and involve qualified nutrition experts (e.g. dietitians) who can advise on suitable alternative foods to prevent depletion of essential nutrients.

Food Safety

Food safety is an issue that has attracted huge public debate within the media, particularly in relation to genetically modified foods. It is important that health professionals provide unbiased and accurate information in this field to enable consumers to make their own choices about the foods they wish to eat.

Q5.14 What are genetically modified foods?

Genetically modified (GM) foods are foods that have had their genotype modified by the technological introduction, or deletion, of genetic information. There are potential advantages to these types of foods, particularly in terms of increasing the efficiency of food production and the variety of foods available on the market. There are also a number of concerns about implementing this type of technology. In particular, there has been massive coverage in the media, which has raised concerns over the safety of GM food and the impact on the environment. For a brief review of the situation, see Pickard (1999).

Individual characteristics of a plant, such as the height to which it grows, its ability to resist disease or the colour of its petals, are determined by its genes. These characteristics, or traits, are inherited from generation to generation. GM technology involves copying the genes that govern a particular characteristic from one plant and transferring them to another. Similar techniques are used in conventional plant breeding, but in this case traits can be transferred only between plants (or between animals, e.g. cattle) of the same or closely related species. Genetic modification enables traits to be transferred between different species, and potentially even between animals and plants. For example, 'Bt maize' has been genetically modified to make it produce a protein (from the bacterium *Bacillus thuringiensis*) that kills the corn borer insect, which can be a major threat to maize crops. Other traits that could be introduced include improved nutritional value (e.g. higher iron content in rice) and the ability to survive in drought, flood or frost conditions.

In discussion about the impact of GM technology, it is often forgotten that the conventionally grown crops that we eat today are very different from their wild ancestors, which have been modified over the centuries by selective breeding techniques, to produce higher yields, for example.

The long-term consequences of using GM technology in food production are largely unknown. It is very important, therefore, that sufficient research is undertaken before these foods are made available to the consumer, and that the impact on the environment is constantly monitored.

Whether or not the public will accept GM technology very much depends on their confidence in the regulatory process. Currently, GM crops are subject to a number of stringent regulatory hurdles. First, the genetic modification is thoroughly tested in the laboratory, often for a number of years, to check that there are no adverse consequences. This is regulated by an EU Directive which is implemented in the UK as the Genetically Modified Organisms (contained use) Regulations. Those wishing to carry out tests have to register with the Health and Safety Executive. If these tests are passed, producers may wish to conduct a field trial. These are governed by yet another EU Directive and anyone wishing to conduct such a trial has to apply to the Department of the Environment, Transport and the Regions. All applications are comprehensively reviewed by the Advisory Committee on Releases to the Environment (ACRE), membership of which includes experts in ecology, biodiversity and farming practice.

At the time of writing, no GM crops are being grown commercially in the UK, but this crucial step would involve further review by both UK and EU expert committees, including ACNFP (the UK Government's Advisory Committee on Novel Foods and Processes) and COT (the Government's Committee on Toxicity of Chemicals in Food, Consumer Products and the Environment).

Foods available, at the time of writing, that have been produced using GM technology have successfully passed the regulatory hurdles described above and so can be regarded as perfectly safe to eat. These include some soya beans, some vegetarian cheeses, some tomatoes and some maize.

Legislation exists to ensure that all foods that contain ingredients derived using GM technology are appropriately labelled to indicate this fact.

The Food and Drink Federation, through its Food Futures Programme, has produced a range of useful publications on this important topic (see Useful addresses).

Q5.15 What about organic foods?

Organic production systems are designed to produce foods of high nutritional quality by using systems that aim to avoid the use of pesticides and that have minimum effect on the environment and on wildlife, e.g. via the choice of fertiliser.

It is worth noting, however, that pesticides are used to keep food disease-free and levels of pesticide residues on conventionally produced fruit and vegetables are very low, if present at all. These low levels do not present a risk to human health. All pesticides have been thoroughly tested for their effects on health and levels are constantly monitored.

In 1997, 70% of food samples analysed by MAFF for their pesticide residue content were found to be residue free; 29% contained levels below the maximum residue level (MRL). The MRL is the maximum level expected to be found in a sample and is the legal standard against which residues are measured. The MRL is not the same as the acceptable daily intake (ADI). Even if people were to consume large amounts of foods containing the MRL, they would not be expected to reach the ADI, because a large margin of safety has been incorporated. The ADI takes into account vulnerable groups such as children and elderly people.

There is no evidence to show that fruit and vegetables grown organically have a better nutrient content than those produced non-organically. All fruit and vegetables, whatever their origin, should be washed or peeled as appropriate before consumption: this is standard hygienic practice to counteract contamination with dust and other foreign particles likely to be encountered during storage and transportation. Organic vegetables tend to be relatively expensive and for this reason it would be irresponsible to recommend organic produce only, because this may detrimentally affect the diet of those members of the population who have less money to spend on food. It is important to encourage everybody to eat a wide variety of fruit and vegetables from whatever origin. The consumption of organic produce is a matter of individual choice.

One of the facets of organic farming is the use of a different range of fertilisers. The use of animal waste as fertiliser, whether in producing organic or non-organic food, may pose a risk of contamination with pathogens, and consequent food poisoning from foods that are consumed raw or with inadequate cooking. Fruit and vegetables, in particular, whether organic or non-organic, should be washed thoroughly if they are to be consumed raw.

> Q5.16 What guidance should be offered to the public to reduce the risks of
> food poisoning resulting from poor food handling in the home?

In recent years, there have been concerns about the increase in reported cases of food-borne infection. Figure 5.1 shows the substantial increase that has occurred in food poisoning over the 15-year period from 1982 to 1997. The Government has recently set up a Food Standards Agency; part of the remit of this agency will be to provide independent and authoritative advice to the public on food safety. The Food Standards Bill to put these proposals into effect was introduced to Parliament in June 1999, and the Agency came into being in April 2000.

In particular, there has been an increase in cases of infection with *Campylobacter* over the last few years, whereas *Salmonella* infections are on the decline. The latest food poisoning statistics indicate that, of the 100 000 reported cases, 58 000 are caused by *Campylobacter* and 23 000 are a result of *Salmonella* infection. The Government has estimated that, for every reported case of infection with *Campylobacter*, eight further cases go unreported.

Number of reports (thousands)

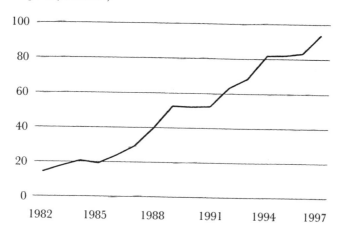

(Source: Public Health Laboratory Service. Crown copyright material is produced with the permission of the controller of Her Majesty's Stationery Office.)

Figure 5.1 The rising trend of reports of food poisoning. England and Wales 1997 data are provisional.

Good hygienic practices in the home when preparing, cooking and storing food will help ensure that the food consumed is wholesome and fit to eat. Guidelines for good hygienic practices in the home are shown in Box 5.1, see page 184. For further information on food poisoning and infection control see Duggal, Jenkinson and Beaumont, Infection Control: A Handbook for Community Nurses in this series.

Box 5.1 General guidelines on cleanliness in the kitchen

Keep all work surfaces scrupulously clean
Wash all cooking utensils after they have come into contact with raw meat, poultry
    or eggs to prevent cross-contamination
Use separate chopping boards for foods that are to be cooked, e.g. raw meat
Keep kitchen cloths clean
Rinse crockery in hot water, leave to dry, then wipe clean with a tea towel
Use kitchen paper towel to mop up spills, rather than a dishcloth
Keep waste bins covered and away from food
Keep pets away from the kitchen.

Hygienic food handling
Wash all equipment and work surfaces before and after touching raw food
Wash all foods that are to be eaten raw thoroughly
Cook meat thoroughly to an internal temperature of at least 70°C
When cooking rolled meats, sausages and burgers, check that the juices run clear
    and no pink bits remain
When using a microwave to reheat food, observe the standing times recommended
    by the manufacturer to ensure that the food attains an even temperature before it
    is eaten
Keep raw and cooked foods separate during preparation and storage
Cool cooked foods as quickly as possible if they are to be stored
Always cover foods and do not leave standing around in the kitchen
Store food at the correct temperature (< 4°C in the fridge or < −18°C in the freezer).
    A thermometer may be useful to ensure that the temperatures are correct
Store raw meat, well covered, at the bottom of the fridge
Store eggs in the fridge, if possible
Never overload the fridge because this can reduce the circulation of cool air
Keep foods for as short a time as possible (especially meat and fish) and follow stor-
    age instructions. Do not use beyond the 'use by' or 'best before' date
Thaw frozen meat thoroughly before cooking
Avoid re-heating any food more than once
If food is re-heated, do so thoroughly.

Personal hygiene
Always wash hands thoroughly before preparing food, after visiting the toilet and
    after emptying the rubbish bin
Never lick fingers or utensils and put them back into food
Wash hands after blowing your nose while handling food
Keep nails clean and hair out of food
Wear a clean apron
Do not handle food if you have a heavy cold, sickness or diarrhoea
Cover all cuts, spots and pimples, particularly on the hands, with a waterproof dress-
    ing and replace it often.

Q5.17 Is it true that malnutrition in hospitals is on the increase?

There is growing concern about the poor nutritional status of many people entering hospital, particularly those with chronic disease. It is estimated that 40% of adults and 15% of children are malnourished on admission to hospital. This can influence both the outcome of their disease and the length of their stay. Undernutrition is often unrecognised and untreated in hospital patients, many of whom continue to lose weight while in hospital, reflecting the inadequacy of current feeding policies. Malnutrition in hospitals is not a new problem; it is unfortunately an on-going, complex problem, which has roots in each link of the food chain from hospital kitchen to patient's mouth. A recent report has suggested that between 30% and 40% of the food provided in hospitals is thrown away and average food intakes are less than 75% of that recommended, particularly among elderly people (BAPEN, 1999). This impairs clinical outcome and wastes resources. An article on this topic and a summary of a conference addressing these issues can be found in two recent issues of *Nutrition Bulletin* (Schenker, 1999, 2000).

The Malnutrition Advisory Group (MAG) has recently developed a tool for assessing the presence of undernutrition, using measurements of height and weight, and information about recent weight change (Malnutrition Advisory Group, 2000) (see Useful Addresses).

Chapter 6
Assessing the Quality of Nutritional Information

This chapter briefly examines the importance of assessing the validity of new research, to enable the reader to understand the value of reports. The role of dietetic/nutrition specialists is outlined.

Assessing the Validity of New Research

Q6.1 Can the source of the paper give some indication of its validity?

The result of any published work is only as good as its design methodology. It is therefore important to consider the quality of the data presented in any scientific paper before accepting its findings and applying these to your own patients or clients. The source of the paper can provide an indication of its likely validity. A paper that is published in a peer-reviewed journal has been sent to experts in the field, who have agreed that this paper is of a sufficient standard to be published in that particular journal. Nevertheless, the review process is not perfect and studies with weak methodology do get published in highly respected journals. It is therefore essential to have some understanding of how to determine whether the results of a paper can be relied upon. This section provides some guidance on how to assess the reliability and validity of a scientific paper.

Q6.2 What are the main questions to ask when reading a paper?

The results of a research study will depend on the question that the study is asking and how it is being asked. Certain key questions must therefore be considered when reading any scientific paper (Box 6.1)

Box 6.1 The main questions to ask when reading a paper

What was the objective of the study?

What was the study design and was it appropriate to address the objectives of the study?

What was the study group and how was it selected?

Were the measurements likely to be valid and reliable?

Were other factors that might be related to the exposure and outcome of interest measured?

Are the data adequately described?

How should the findings be interpreted?

How do the results compare with previous reports?

What are the implications of the study?

What was the objective of the study?

All scientific papers should have the purpose of the study clearly stated in the introduction section. This suggests that the research hypothesis was specified in advance, resulting in a well-planned study. In contrast, the absence of any statement indicates that the authors themselves were not clear about what they were trying to find out. This may have provided an opportunity to trawl though the results, looking for any significant relationship, which makes it likely that spurious results may have been obtained.

What was the study design and was it appropriate to address the objectives of the study?

The methods section of any paper provides essential information about who was studied and how the study was carried out, and is a vital guide to the quality of a paper. The first factor to consider is the type of study that has been conducted and whether this is appropriate to address the objectives of the study.

To determine the link between nutrients and disease in humans, we cannot rely on molecular and animal studies. Nutritional epidemiological studies must be performed to provide information about the relationship between nutrition and health in human populations consuming usual amounts of foods and nutrients. Such studies aim to explore the relationship between what people eat (the exposure) and health (the outcome), which can be assessed either as increased risk of disease (e.g. a high cholesterol level) or presence of disease (e.g. a heart attack). The main purpose is to identify causes so that these can be altered in order to reduce the health burden. For a dietary factor to be the cause of ill-health, it must be demonstrated to occur before the onset of an illness or disease, and its effect must not be the result of a chance association or some other factor (such as a confounder). Causality can be tested only in a carefully controlled experiment where the exposure is changed and everything else held constant, and the effects on the outcome are measured with complete accuracy. An experimental study attempts to do this. A clinical trial or randomised controlled trial is a controlled experiment in which the investigator changes only one dietary factor and looks at the effect on the outcome of interest. In many circumstances, this type of approach is not, however, possible and most studies are observational – the investigator does not intervene but simply assesses the differences in the exposure and outcome of interest to see whether the two might be related. Although such studies cannot provide evidence of causality, they can be used by researchers to identify dietary factors that might be involved in the onset of disease.

There are four main types of observational study:

1. An ecological study compares patterns of disease in different populations or groups with very different diets, e.g. this type of study might measure the average amount of fat in the diet in populations and relate this to their incidence of coronary heart disease.
2. A cross-sectional study investigates individuals, rather than populations, and measures both the outcome and the exposure at the same time, without prior knowledge of either, e.g. a study may measure the amount of fat in the diet of individuals and their cholesterol levels at the same time point.
3. A case–control study compares past exposure to a dietary factor between groups of individuals with and without the disease of interest, e.g. people with heart disease may be asked about their past fat intake and this is compared with information from individuals matched for criteria such as age, sex, smoking habits, blood pressure, etc.
4. A cohort (or prospective) study measures the exposure of interest in a group of individuals and follows this group over time recording the incidence of the outcome of interest, e.g. a study might

assess fat intake in a group of individuals and follow them over time to compare heart disease rates. Dietary measurements are usually made at several points during the follow-up period. An example of a cohort study is the US Nurses Study conducted at Harvard.

Each study design has advantages and disadvantages. The primary problem of ecological studies, comparing different populations, is that there are many potential determinants of disease other than the dietary factor under consideration, which may vary in prevalence between areas of the world with a high or a low incidence of disease. These include genetic predisposition, other dietary factors, environmental factors and lifestyle practices. In cross-sectional studies of individuals, both the dietary factor and the disease, or risk of disease, are measured at the same time. It is therefore not possible to assess whether any difference in diet occurred before, or as a consequence of, the disease. Another problem for this study design is that current diet may not be the most appropriate measure, e.g. people who are aware that they have high cholesterol levels may have already changed their diet. Recalling past diet is not very reliable. This is also a problem for case–control studies. Recall bias can also occur because subjects who know that they have an illness are more likely to recall the exposure. This would give an erroneous relationship between exposure and disease.

Cohort (prospective) studies do not have this problem and their findings are generally considered to be more reliable. However, such studies are expensive and take a long time. They cannot be performed for rare diseases because an excessive amount of time would be required before any cases of the disease occurred within the study population. For this reason, cohort studies often rely on surrogate markers (such as cholesterol levels as an indicator of heart disease risk). The problems presented by each design must be considered when assessing the validity of a study and how its results may be generalised to other populations or circumstances. For those particularly interested in systematic review, a method for scoring case–control and cohort studies has been developed by Margetts et al. (1995) and was in fact used in assessment of the data on diet and cancer by the Government advisory committee, COMA (Department of Health, 1998c).

What was the study group and how was it selected?

A scientific paper must provide sufficient information about who was studied and how they were recruited. Such information is necessary in order to assess how widely the results of any study can be generalised to other circumstances. It is also essential to estimate the risk of bias, which can cause misleading results and lead to incorrect conclusions. Bias can arise both in the way the subjects are selected and/or when the data are being collected. Key factors to consider include the inclusion and exclusion criteria used to determine who takes part in the study and whether the subjects were volunteers or a representative sample of a larger group.

In any study, there is also the possibility of chance affecting the findings. Sometimes what looks like an interesting result could be a statistical fluke. A study with lots of people is less likely to be influenced by chance and the size of the sample studied is therefore extremely important. For example, in a sample of 10 babies we would expect half of them to be girls and half boys but would not be surprised to find seven girls and three boys. However, if we took a sample of 1000, we would be unlikely to find 700 girls and 300 boys. The authors of any paper should justify their choice of sample size in the methods section. A formal sample size calculation is usually carried out to determine how big the sample should be to detect any relevant effect.

Are the measurements likely to be valid and reliable?

Poor measuring techniques can lead to substantial errors. The circumstances in which the measurements of both the dietary factor and the disease or risk factor were made should be described, together with the steps taken to ensure the accuracy of these measurements. For example, if a questionnaire was used to assess dietary intake of a food or nutrient, this should be piloted and tested beforehand, to ensure that it measured what it should be measuring (valid) and would find the same results if used more than once (reliable). The measurement of dietary exposure is very difficult. Any method will involve some error (measurement error), but the size of this error will vary depending on the method used. It is therefore necessary to look at how it is done and make a judgement about its likely accuracy. What is important is whether any error is likely to be related in any way to the exposure or outcome of interest. If it is, this will cause bias in the results and lead to misinterpretation. Misleading information can also be collected when patients have to remember past events because their recall can be influenced by many other factors, e.g. the need to find an explanation for their disease. This is a common problem in case–control studies. Several studies will discuss the likelihood of measurement error in the discussion section.

Were other factors that might be related to the exposure and outcome of interest measured?

To determine whether a dietary factor can cause a disease, it is necessary to ensure that any relationship between the two is not the result of some other factor (a confounder). Confounding occurs because many aspects of human health and behaviour are interrelated. This arises when part of the observed relationship between an exposure and an outcome is the result of the action of another factor that is directly related to both. For example, the consumption of alcohol will be related to lung cancer because both are related to smoking and it is smoking that causes lung cancer. It is therefore necessary to think about all potential confounding factors, and to ensure that these have been measured and their effects considered in the interpretation of the study results.

Are the data adequately described?

Data should be laid out in a logical fashion and clearly presented. The main findings of most studies are usually presented in the form of tables and figures. The text of the results section should lead the reader through these data and highlight key facts. The statistical methods used should also be described. This information is necessary to allow the reader to judge whether the information is accurate.

How should the findings be interpreted?

The authors' conclusions about the results of their study cannot always be relied upon because researchers can be more enthusiastic about their findings than is strictly warranted. The key findings should therefore be assessed by the reader in relation to any defects in the design, conduct or analysis of the study. It is therefore important to assess the risk of bias and confounding in the study. The size of any reported effect must be considered to see whether it is likely to be of clinical importance. Findings can be considered to be more valid when there is evidence of a dose–response (i.e. a high exposure carries a greater risk than a lesser one) and when they are biologically plausible. Interpreting the findings of a study requires judgement and can be improved with experience.

How do the results compare with previous reports?

The findings of a single study are unlikely to provide convincing evidence. New findings are usually accepted only when they are supported by a substantial body of research, using different study designs and derived from several research groups. Therefore the findings of any study should be interpreted in the light of previous reports and any discrepancies addressed.

What are the implications of the study?

Several factors must be considered in order to determine whether the results of a study should lead to changes in the management of one's own patients/clients. The first important question is whether the size of the effect is of clinical importance. Second, the quality of the study must be considered and its findings compared with evidence from previous reports, in order to determine whether the results are likely to be reliable. Last, whether the results can be applied to your patients will be determined by how far the results can be generalised to other times, locations, populations or age groups. This assessment can be subjective and must be done with caution. How similar the patients studied are to yours, and whether the conditions in which the study was carried out resemble local conditions, will indicate whether the same size of effect is likely to occur in your patients.

Who to Approach for Detailed Professional Nutritional Advice

Q6.3 What does a dietitian do and how do I obtain a referral to a dietitian?

A state-registered dietitian will have undertaken training in both hospital and community settings as part of his or her course, and is qualified to give practical advice to individuals about their diets.

Most dietitians are employed in the NHS, and they work with both healthy and sick people, as well as the families of these. With patients who need special diets, dietitians use their scientific knowledge to provide practical information that is appropriate to the patient's medical history and lifestyle. State-registered dietitians will have the letters SRD after their name. For a dietitian in the NHS to give advice to a patient, a referral must be obtained, either from a hospital doctor or from the patient's GP. However, there are also freelance state-registered dietitians.

Further information on the role of state-registered dietitians and how they can be contacted can be obtained from the British Dietetic Association (see Useful Addresses).

Q6.4 What does the title registered public health nutritionist (RPHNutr) mean?

Public health nutrition is the application of the science of nutrition for the benefit of the population as a whole, or subsections of the population. It encompasses promotion of good health through nutrition and the primary prevention of diet-related illness in the population. Although an important facet of public health nutrition is establishing the relationships between nutrition and health or disease risk at a research level, equally important is nutrition-related health promotion. This includes the type of work conducted by many of the nutritionists working in Government, and in the food industry and related trade associations, by dietitians working in the community, and by nutritionists engaged in local health promotion.

In December 1997, the Nutrition Society launched a scheme to register individuals qualified in public health nutrition. Registration usually requires a university degree in human nutrition plus a minimum of 3 years relevant postgraduate experience in public health nutrition. Individuals achieving registration are known as registered public health nutritionists (RPHNutr after their name). The Nutrition Society is also beginning to accredit degree courses in public health nutrition, so that this career path can be selected from the outset. Some accredited courses are already available. Further details can be obtained from the Nutrition Society's website (www.nutsoc.org.uk).

References

Abel EL (1998). *Fetal Alcohol Syndrome Revisited*. New York: Plenum Press.

Abrams B, Duncan D, Hertz-Picciotto J (1993). A prospective study of dietary intake and acquired deficiency syndrome in HIV-seropositive homosexual men. *J AIDS* 6: 949–58.

Acheson D (1998). *Independent Inquiry into Inequalities in Health Report*. London: The Stationery Office.

Albertazzi P, Pansini F, Bottazzi M, Bonaccorsi G, De Aloysio D, Morton MS (1999). Dietary soy supplementation and phytoestrogen levels. *Obstet Gynecol* 94: 229–31.

Barker ME, McClean SI, Thompson KA, Reid NG (1990). Dietary behaviours and sociological demographics in Northern Ireland. *Br J Nutr* 64: 319–29.

Barker DJP (1992). *Fetal and Infant Origins of Adult Disease*. London: BMJ Publishing Group.

Baum M, Cassetti L, Bonvehi P, Shor-Posner G, Lu Y, Sauberlich H (1994). Inadequate dietary intake and altered nutrition status in early HIV-1 infection. *Nutrition* 10: 116–20.

Berenson GS, Srinivasan SR, Bao W (1997). Precursors of cardiovascular risk in young adults from a biracial (black-white) population: the Bogalusa Heart Study. *Ann N Y Acad Sci* 817: 189–98.

BAPEN (1999). A Report by a Working Party of the British Association for Parenteral and Enteral Nutrition. *Hospital Food as Treatment*. Allison SP, ed. Kent: BAPEN.

British Heart Foundation (1998). *Coronary Heart Disease Statistics*. Oxford: British Heart Foundation.

British Nutrition Foundation (1992). *Coronary Heart Disease – 2. What is it and what are the uncontrollable factors?* Briefing paper 28. London: British Nutrition Foundation.

British Nutrition Foundation (1993). *Diet and Heart Disease: A round table of factors*. Ashwell M, ed. Briefing paper. London: British Nutrition Foundation.

British Nutrition Foundation (1995). *Vegetarianism*. Briefing paper. London: British Nutrition Foundation.

British Nutrition Foundation (1997). *Nutrition in Infancy*. Briefing paper. London: British Nutrition Foundation.

British Nutrition Foundation (1999a). *Obesity. The Report of the British Nutrition Foundation Task Force*. London: Blackwell Science.

British Nutrition Foundation Task Force on Oral Health (1999b). *Diet and Other Factors. The Report of the British Nutrition Foundation Task Force*. The Netherlands: Elsevier Science BV.

British Nutrition Foundation (1999c). *n-3 Fatty Acids and Health*. Briefing Paper. London: British Nutrition Foundation.

British Nutrition Foundation (2000). *Food Allergy and Intolerance*. Briefing Paper. London: British Nutrition Foundation.

British Nutrition Foundation (2001a). *Selenium and Health*. Briefing Paper. London: British Nutrition Foundation.

British Nutrition Foundation (2001b). *Nutrition and Sport*. Briefing Paper. London: British Nutrition Foundation.

Bull NL (1985). Dietary habits of 15 to 25 year olds. *Human Nutrition: Applied Nutrition* 39A(suppl 1): 1–68.

Burr ML, Fehily AM, Gilbert JF et al. (1989). Effects of changes in fat, fish and fibre intakes on death and myocardial reinfarction: Diet and Reinfarction Trial (DART). *Lancet* ii: 757–61.

Buttriss J (1999). Nutrition in older people – the public health message. *Nutrition Bulletin* 24: 48–57.

Buttriss J (2000a). Is Britain ready for FOSHU? *Nutrition Bulletin* 25: 159–61.

Buttriss J (2000b). Diet and nutritional status of 4–18 year olds – public health implications. *BNF Nutrition Bulletin* 25: 209–17.

Buttriss J, Bundy R, Hughes J (2000). An update on vitamin K: contribution of MAFF-funded research. *Nutrition Bulletin* 25: 125–34.

Cann CE, Martin MC, Genant HK, Jaffe PB (1984). Decreased spinal mineral content in amenorrheic women. *JAMA* 251: 626–29.

Caroline Walker Trust (1995). *Eating Well for Older People*. London: Caroline Walker Trust.

Cassidy A, Bingham S, Setchell KD (1994) Biological effects of a diet of soy protein rich in isoflavones on the menstrual cycle of premenopausal women. *Am J Clin Nutr* 60: 333–40.

Catassi C, Ratsch IM, Fabiani E (1994) Coeliac disease in the year (2000): exploring the iceberg. *Lancet* 343: 200–3.

Chaturvedi N, McKeigue PM, Marmot MG (1993). Resting and ambulatory blood pressure differences in Afro-Caribbeans and Europeans. *Hypertension* 22: 90–6.

Cieslik W, Jones S, Atton C (1999). Health needs of young people: Eating disorders. In: *The Informed Practice Nurse*. Edwards M, ed. London: Whurr Publishers.

Committee on Toxicity (COT) (1997). *Statement on Vitamin B₆ (Pyridoxine) Toxicity*. London: Department of Health.

Committee on Toxicity of Chemicals in Food, Consumer Products and the Environment (2000). *Adverse Reactions to Food and Food Ingredients*. London: Food Standards Agency.

Crawley H (1993). Plan before conception for a healthy pregnancy. *MIMS* 19 Jan: 24–9.

Crouse JR (1989). Gender, lipoproteins, diet and cardiovascular risk. *Lancet* 336: 474–81.

De Lorgeril M, Renaud S, Mamelle N et al. (1994). Mediterranean alpha-linolenic acid-rich diet in secondary prevention of coronary heart disease. *Lancet* 343: 1454–9.

Department for Education and Employment (2000a). *The Education (Nutritional Standards for School Lunches) (England)) Regulations*. London: The Stationery Office.

Department for Education and Employment (2000b). *Guidance for Caterers on Implementing National Nutritional Standards for Healthy School Lunches (2000)*. London: The Stationery Office.

Department of Health (1991). *Dietary Reference Values for Food Energy and Nutrients for the UK. Report on Health and Social Subjects*, No. 41. London: HMSO.

Department of Health (1992). *The Health of the Nation. A Strategy for Health in England.* London: HMSO.

Department of Health (1994a). *Eat Well!: An Action Plan from the Nutrition Task Force to Achieve the Health of the Nation Targets on Diet and Nutrition.* London: HMSO.

Department of Health (1994b). *Nutritional Aspects of Cardiovascular Disease. Report on Health and Social Subjects*, No. 46. London: HMSO.

Department of Health (1994c). *Weaning and the Weaning Diet. Report on Health and Social Subjects*, No. 45. London: HMSO.

Department of Health (1995a). *Sensible Drinking. The Report of an Inter-Departmental Working Group.* London: Department of Health.

Department of Health (1995b*). The Health of the Nation. More People More Active More Often: Physical Activity in England. A Consultative Paper.* London: HMSO.

Department of Health (1996a). *Health Survey for England 1994.* London: HMSO.

Department of Health (1996b). *Low Income, Food, Nutrition and Health: Strategies for Improvement.* London: Department of Health.

Department of Health (1998). *Committee on Toxicity of Chemicals in Food, Consumer Products and the Environment. Peanut Allergy.* London: Department of Health.

Department of Health (1998a). *Nutrition and Bone Health. Report on Health and Social Subjects*, No. 49. London: The Stationery Office.

Department of Health (1998b). *Health Survey for England 1996.* London: The Stationery Office.

Department of Health (1998c). *Nutritional Aspects of the Development of Cancer. Report on Health and Social Subjects*, No. 48. London: The Stationery Office.

Department of Health (1998d). *Health Survey for England. The Health of Young People '95–'97.* London: The Stationery Office.

Department of Health (1999). *Saving Lives: Our Healthier Nation.* London: The Stationery Office.

Department of Health (2000a). *The NHS Plan.* London: The Stationery Office.

Department of Health (2000b). *The NHS Cancer Plan.* London: Department of Health.

Department of Health (2000c). *National Service Framework for Coronary Heart Disease.* London: Department of Health.

Department of Health (2000d). *Folic Acid and the Prevention of Disease. Report on Health and Social Subjects.* London: The Stationery Office.

Department of Health and Social Security (1980). *Inequalities in Health: Report of a Research Working Group.* London: DHSS.

Department of Health and Social Security (1989). *The Diets of British Schoolchildren. Report on Health and Social Subjects*, 36. London: HMSO.

Diabetes UK (2000) http://www.diabetes.org.uk.

Doll H, Brown S, Thurston A, Vessey M (1989). Pyridoxine (vitamin B_6) and the premenstrual syndrome: a randomized controlled crossover trial. *J R Coll Gen Practit* 39: 364–8.

Eating Disorders Association (1995). *Eating Disorders – A Guide for Primary Care.* Norwich: Eating Disorders Association.

Edwards M (1996). Silent suffering. *Practice Nurse* 12: 628–30.

Ernhart CB, Sokol RJ, Martier S et al. (1987). Alcohol teratogenicity in the human: a detailed assessment of specificity, critical period, and threshold. *Am J Obstet Gynecol* 156: 33–9.

Finch S, Doyle W, Lowe C et al. (1998). *National Diet and Nutrition Survey: People aged 65 Years and Over.* London: HMSO.

Forster D, Pannell D, Edwards M (1999). Health promotion: promoting preconception care. In: *The Informed Practice Nurse.* Edwards M, ed. London: Whurr Publishers.

Gaby SK, Bendich A, Singh VN, Machlin LJ (1991). *Vitamin Intake and Health: A Scientific Review.* New York: Marcel Dekker Inc.

Gardner Merchant School Meals Survey (1998). *What are Today's Children Eating?* Surrey: Gardner Merchant.

German JB (1999). Butyric acid in cancer prevention. *Nutrition Bulletin* 24: 203–9.

GISSI-Prevenzione Investigators (1999). Dietary supplementation with n-3 polyunsaturated fatty acids and vitamin E after myocardial infarction: results of the GISSI-Prevenzione trial. *Lancet* 354: 447–55.

Gregory JR, Hinds K (1995). *National Diet and Nutrition Survey of Children Aged 1.5–4.5 Years. Report of the Dental Survey,* Volume 2. London: HMSO.

Gregory J, Foster K, Tyler H, Wiseman M (1990). *The Dietary and Nutritional Survey of British Adults.* London: HMSO.

Gregory J, Collins D, Davies P, Hughes J, Clarke P (1995). *National Diet and Nutrition Survey. Children aged 1.5 to 4.5 years.* London: HMSO.

Gregory J, Lowe S, Bates CJ et al. (2000). *National Diet and Nutrition Survey: Young People aged 4 to 18 years,* Volume 1: *Report of the diet and nutrition survey.* London: The Stationery Office.

Hanes FA, De Looy AE (1987). Can I afford the diet? *Hum Nutr Appl Nutr* 41: 1–12.

Health Education Authority (1995). *The Balance of Good Health.* London: Department for Education and Employment.

Høst A (1997). Cow's milk allergy. *J R Soc Med* 90(suppl 30): 34–9.

Howlett M, McClelland L, Crisp AH (1995). The cost of the illness that defies. *Postgrad Med J* 71: 36–9.

Hughes J, Buttriss J (2000). An update on folates and folic acid: contribution of MAFF-funded research. *Nutrition Bulletin* 25: 113–24.

Institute of Grocery Distribution (1998). *Voluntary Nutrition Labelling Guidelines to Benefit the Consumer.* Watford: Institute of Grocery Distribution.

Johnston SD, Watson RG, McMillan SA, Sloan J, Love AH (1998). Coeliac disease detected by screening is not silent – simply unrecognised. *Q J Med* 91: 853–60.

Kannel WB, Ellison RC (1996). Alcohol and coronary heart disease: the evidence for a protective effect. *Clin Chim Acta* 246: 59–76.

Lawrence RA (1989). Drugs in breast milk and the effect on the infant. In: *Breast-Feeding: A Guide for the Medical Profession.* Lawrence RA, ed. 3rd edn. St Louis: CV Mosby Co.

MacDonald A (1995). Which formula in cows milk protein intolerance? *Eur J Clin Nutr* 49(suppl 1): 56–63.

Malnutrition Advisory Group (2000) *Screening Tool for Adults at Risk of Malnutrition.* London: BAPEN (www.bapen.org.uk).

McKeigue PM, Shah B, Marmot MG (1991). Relation of central obesity and insulin resistance with high diabetes prevalence and cardiovascular risk in South asians. *Lancet* 337: 382–6.

Margetts B, Thompson RL, Key T et al. (1995). Development of a scoring system to judge the scientific quality of information from case-control and cohort studies of nutrition and disease. *Nutr Cancer* 24: 231–9.

Mather HM, Keen H (1985). The Southall diabetes survey: Prevalence of known diabetes in Asians and Europeans. *BMJ* 291: 1081–4.

Ministry of Agriculture, Fisheries and Food (1998a). *Fatty Acids*. Supplement to McCance and Widdowson's *The Composition of Foods* (7th Supplement). London: Royal Society of Chemistry.

Ministry of Agriculture, Fisheries and Food (1998b). *Report of the Review of MAFF's Food Intolerance Research Programme*, Chief Scientist's Group. London: MAFF.

Ministry of Agriculture, Fisheries and Food (1999) *National Food Survey 1998*. London: The Stationery Office.

Ministry of Agriculture, Fisheries and Foods (2000). *National Food Survey 1999*. London: The Stationery Office.

MRC Vitamin Study Group (1991). Prevention of neural tube defects: results of the Medical Research Council Vitamin Study. *Lancet* 238: 131–7.

National Academy of Sciences Food and Nutrition Board (1990). *Sub-committee on Nutritional Status and Weight Gain during Pregnancy*. Washington DC: National Academy Press.

National Dairy Council (1989). *Nutrition and Teenagers*. London: NDC.

National Dairy Council (1990). *Teenage Eating Habits and Attitudes to Food*. London: NDC.

National Dairy Council (1998). *Adverse Reactions to Food*. Topical Update – 2. London: NDC.

National Health Service Executive (1999). *Making a Difference*. London: The Stationery Office.

Nicholl CG, Levy JC, Rao PV, Mather HM (1986). Asian diabetes in Britain: a clinical profile. *Diabetic Med* 3: 257–60.

Not T, Horvath K, Hill ID et al. (1998) Coeliac disease in the USA: high prevalence of antiendoysium antibodies in healthy blood donors. *Scand J Gastroenterol* 33: 494–8.

O'Brien M (1994). *Children's dental health in the United Kingdom*. London: OPCS.

Pickard R (1999). Genetically modified foods – science in retreat. *The Biochemist* October: 32–3.

Prescott-Clarke P, Primatesta P, eds (1998). *Health Survey for England 1996*. London: The Stationery Office.

Ranjan V (1993). Pregnancy in the under 16's: waking up to the realities. *Professional Care of Mother and Child* 3(2): 34–5.

Realeat (1993). *Changing Attitudes to Meat Consumption*. London: Realeat.

Rees JM, Mahan LK (1988). Nutrition in adolescence. In: *Nutrition Throughout the Life Cycle* Williams SR, Worthington-Roberts BS, eds. St Louis: Times Mirror/Mosby College Publishing.

Rees GA, Trevan M, Davies GJ (1994). Dietary fibre modification and the symptoms of irritable bowel syndrome – a review. *J Hum Nutr Diet* 7: 179–89.

Rivers JM (1975). Oral contraceptives and ascorbic acid. *Am J Clin Nutr* 28: 550–4.

Rosado JL (1997). Lactose digestion and maldigestion: implications for dietary habits in developing countries. *Nutr Res Rev* 5: 203–23.

Royal College of Psychiatrists (1992). *Eating Disorders*. Council Report CR14. London: RCPsych.

Shepherd R, Paisley CM, Sparks P, Anderson AS, Eley S, Lean MEJ (1996). Constraints on dietary choice: the role of income. *Nutr Food Sci* 5: 19–21.

Schenker S (1999). Malnutrition in hospital. *Nutrition Bulletin* 24: 131–6.

Schenker S. (2000). Malnutrition in the UK. *Nutrition Bulletin* 25: 175–8.

SI 1499 (1996). *The Food Labelling Regulations of 1996*. London: HMSO.

Smithers G, Gregory JR, Bates CJ, Prentice A, Jackson LV, Wenlock R (2000). The National Diet and Nutrition Survey: young people aged 4–18 years. *Nutrition Bulletin* 25: 105–11.

Steele JG, Sheiham A, Marcenes W, Wallis AWG (1998). *National Diet and Nutrition Survey: People aged 65 years or over. Vol 2: Report of the Oral Health Survey*. London: HMSO.

Stevens-Simon C, McAnarney ER (1988). Adolescent weight gain and low birth weight: a multifactorial model. *Am J Clin Nutr* 47: 948–53.

Stewart AC, Stewart M, Tooley S. (1992). Premenstrual syndrome. Proceedings of a workshop held at the Royal College of Obstetrics and Gynaecologists. London: Medical News Tribute.

The Social Exclusion Unit (1999). *Teenage Pregnancy*. London: The Stationery Office

Tang AM, Graham NM, Kirby AJ, McCall LD, Willett WC, Saah AJ (1993) Dietary micronutrient intake and risk of progression to acquired immunodeficiency syndrome (AIDS) in human imunodeficiency virus type 1 (HIV-1)-infected homosexual men. *Am J Epidemiol* 138: 937–51.

UNAIDS. (1998). *HIV and Infant Feeding. A review of HIV transmission through breastfeeding*. Geneva: World Health Organization.

White A, Freeth S, O'Brien M (1992). *Infant Feeding 1990*. Office of Population Censuses and Surveys. London: HMSO.

World Cancer Research Fund/American Institute for Cancer Research (1997). *Food, Nutrition and the Prevention of Cancer: A global perspective*. Washington DC: WCRF/AICR.

World Health Organization (1982). *Prevention of Coronary Heart Disease*. Technical Report Series No. 678. Geneva: WHO.

Useful addresses

British Dietetic Association
5th Floor, Elizabeth House
22 Suffolk Street
Queensway
Birmingham B1 1LS
Tel: 0121 616 4900
Fax: 0121 616 4901
Website: www.bda.uk.com

British Nutrition Foundation
High Holborn House
52-54 High Holborn
London WC1V 6RQ
Tel: 020 7404 6504
Fax: 020 7404 6747
Website: www.nutrition.org.uk

Child Growth Foundation
2 Mayfield Avenue
Chiswick
London W4 1PW
Tel: 020 8995 0257

Coeliac Society
PO Box 220
High Wycombe
Bucks HP11 2HY
Tel: 01494 437278
Fax: 01494 474349
Website: www.coeliac.co.uk

Diabetes UK (formerly British Diabetes
Association)
10 Queen Anne Street
London W1M 0BD
Tel: 020 7323 1531
Fax: 020 7637 3544
Website: www.diabetes.org.uk

Eating Disorders Association
1st Floor, Wensum House
103 Prince of Wales Road
Norwich
Norfolk NR1 1DW
Helpline: 01603 621414
Youth line: 01603 765050 (4-6pm,
Monday to Friday, 18 years and under)
Fax: 01603 664915
Website: www.edauk.com

Food and Drink Federation
6 Catherine Street
London WC2B 5JJ
Tel: 020 7836 2460
Fax: 020 7836 9757

Institute of Grocery Distribution
Letchmore Heath
Watford
Herts WD2 8QD
Tel: 01923 857141
Fax: 01923 852531
Website: www.igd.org.uk

Food Standards Agency
England
Aviation House
125 Kingsway
London WC2B 6NH
Tel: 020 7276 8000
E-mail:helpline@foodstandards.gsi.gov.uk
Website: www.foodstandards.gov.uk

Scotland
St Magnus House
6th Floor, 25 Guild Street
Aberdeen AB11 6NG
Fax: 01224 285168

Wales
1st Floor, Southgate House
Wood Street
Cardiff CF10 1EW
Fax: 029 2067 8918/8919

Northern Ireland
Annex 4, Castle Buildings
Stormont
Belfast BT4 3SG
Tel: 0845 7573012
Fax: 028 9052 0777

Health Department Agency
Trevelyan House
30 Great Peter Street
London SW1P 2HW
Tel: 020 7413 1873
Website: www.hda–online.org.uk

Sport England
16 Upper Woburn Place
London WC1H 0QP
Website: www.english.sport.gov.uk

Malnutrition Advisory Group (MAG)
10th Floor, 10 Cabot Square
Canary Wharf
London E14 4QB
Tel: 020 7546 1590
Fax: 020 7345 6536
Website: www.bapen.org.uk

Nutrition Society
10 Cambridge Court
210 Shepherds Bush Road
London W6 7NJ
Tel: 020 7602 0228
Fax: 020 7602 1756
Website: www.nutsoc.org.uk

School Nutrition Action Groups
Health Education Trust
18 High Street
Broom, Alcester
Warwickshire B50 4HJ
Fax: 01789 773915
(Please enclose an s.a.e.)

The Anaphylaxis Campaign
2 Clockhouse Road
Farnborough
Hampshire GU14 7QY
Tel: 01252 542029
Website: www.anaphylaxis.org.uk

The National Osteoporosis Society
PO Box 10
Radstock
Bath BA3 3YB
Tel: 01761 471771
Helpline: 01761 472721
Fax: 01761 471104
Website: www.nos.org.uk

National Dairy Council
5-7 John Princes Street
London W1M 0AP
Tel: 020 7499 7822
Fax: 020 7408 1353
Website: www.milk.co.uk

Realeat
Howard Way
Newport Pagnell
Bucks MK16 9PY
Tel: 01908 211311
Fax: 01908 210514
Website: www.haldanefoods.co.uk

Joint Health Claims Initiative
c/o Leatherhead Food RA
Randalls Road
Surrey KT22 7RY
Tel: 01372 822378
Fax: 01372 822288

Sustain Food Poverty Network
94 White Lion Street
London N1 9PF
Tel: 020 7837 1228
Website: www.sustainweb.org

Vegetarian Society
Parkdale, Durham Road
Altrincham
Cheshire WA14 4QG
Tel: 0161 925 2000
Fax: 0161 926 9182
Website: www.vegsoc.org

Index